A Comparative Analysis of the U.K, Canada, and U.S Health Systems

George O. Obikoya

Table of Contents

Executive Summary	3
Introduction	5
U.K Health System in Transition	10
Canada Health System Revisited	43
Fixing the U.S. Health System	80
Conclusion	117

Executive Summary

Health Systems are under scrutiny in the U.K, Canada, and the U.S. The increasing healthcare costs in these countries are eating deeper into their coffers, alarming both governments and the public alike. The call for measures to stop and possibly reverse this trend is becoming louder, and governments in these countries are more than ever keen to do something before it is too late, but what? Health reforms are ongoing exercises in these countries but the problems their health systems confront do not seem to want to go away. Yet, could Canada for example, afford to keep spending over 10% of its Gross Domestic Product (GDP) on healthcare? The National Health Service (NHS) in England will be £ 750m in the red by the end of the FY2005, according to experts, despite its £ 76bn budget. Indeed, although not announced in the recent 2006 (10th) budget by U.K Chancellor of the Exchequer, Gordon Brown, the government plans to infuse an added £6bn into the NHS over the next two years. Meantime, the Royal Free Hospital in London announced on March 22, 2006, that it was cutting 480 jobs and 100 beds in a bid to save £ 25m, part of the over 2,000 job cuts announced at U.K. hospitals in the previous week. Should there not be some way to curtail the increasing healthcare costs, and to enhance the ability of NHS Trusts to deliver qualitative improvements in the health services, to which shorter hospital wait times, for example, would in part point? In the U.S, forecasts for national health spending indicate that it would continue to grow faster than gross domestic product (GDP) between 2003 and 2014 the result, projected increases in health spending as percentages of GDP from 15.3% in 2003 to 18.7% by 2014. Is it any wonder the intense ardor of governments and other healthcare stakeholders to find answers to the country's healthcare problems?

The most important challenges facing health services in these three countries are to reduce soaring healthcare costs and to improve the quality of healthcare delivery, and despite the differences in the funding models of their health systems, they face and need to solve these common problems. The theme of this e-book is an exploration of the solutions to these challenges, applicable to the three health systems, from a healthcare information and communications technologies (ICT) perspective. The e-book discusses the issues and problems peculiar to each health system and explores the commonalities that they share. Employing a process model of healthcare delivery, it analyses the operations of these systems, emphasizing the important role of healthcare ICT as the underlying strand that binds whatever processes operate in tandem to make health systems function. Taking this premise further, the e-book examines specific clinical, administrative, and financial issues, as well as healthcare delivery and health reform models and concepts, revealing their intricacies yet malleability along the continuum of increasing efficiency and effectiveness that interweaving them within a fabric of healthcare ICT could engender. This e-book offers an appraisal of healthcare processes in the three countries in-depth, a detailed review of the various issues and problems that confront their health systems, and a thorough exposition of the possible approaches to addressing their current challenges by exploiting the many opportunities that healthcare ICT offers to improve the operations of their healthcare processes.

Introduction

The oil crisis and recession got most of the blame for the increasing costs of healthcare in most of countries of the Western world in the 1970s through the 1990s. These increases were as much as 36% and 26% of the GDP (Gross Domestic Product, or the total value of goods and services a country produces) in the US and the UK respectively between 1972 and 1982, and 36% and 20% between 1982 and 1992. However, it is doubtful that healthcare costs would have dropped even if recession did not slow GDP growth considering the increasing healthcare needs of the aging population of these countries, among the many other problems facing their health systems. Government foots most of the healthcare bills in many EU countries, in Canada, and indeed in most OECD (Organization of Economic Cooperation and Development) countries, and even in the US, about 45% of the bills. Healthcare reforms are also recurrent activities in these countries, often triggered by concerns about increasing healthcare costs, mediocre public health outcomes, and public sector deficits, among others. There are many other reasons governments embark on healthcare reform, but most of them revolve around healthcare costs, with doctors, some assert, the chief cost drivers, others, medical technology. Questions are beginning to arise regarding the central role physicians play in the allocation of health resources, particularly with regard to their choices of services to patients, including hospitalizations, medications prescribed, lab tests ordered, and so on, and the cost implications of these decisions. Indeed, the call for accountability and more efficient and cost-effective resource allocation continues to boom louder. The public is also interested in the unfolding saga. There is increasing demand for higher quality health services, patient safety, privacy, confidentiality, and security of patient information, and quicker access to care. It is ironical that what many consider misuse of medical technology others attribute to this quest for higher quality driving doctors to recommend unnecessary and costly investigations, in particular also to avoid defensively, litigation for not providing qualitative services. These are among other reasons governments continue to initiate healthcare reforms, which incidentally have emerged in various shapes, forms, and models, including managed care, managed competition reform, internal market reform, and a host of others, and continue to emerge with an increasing focus on the patient, with ideas such as consumer-driven healthcare changing the paradigms of healthcare delivery.

For sure, these various models have their merits and flaws. However, they also have a common denominator, which is to provide better and sustainable health services, and as is now becoming increasingly obvious, a common underlying strand of healthcare information and communications technologies (ICT) crucial to achieving these objectives. Some would insist that physicians do not like outsiders, for example, governments and insurers, "prying" into their professional affairs. There should be no dispute about physicians prerogative on therapeutic modalities, but also precious little about providers of funds used to run health services having the right to demand cost-effective use of the funds, as do indeed, the consumers of healthcare services. It may sound like a somewhat treacherous path to trod trying to find a meeting point between the interests of physicians, providers of healthcare funds, and the public, but it is not nearly that impossible a goal to achieve. It only takes a commitment on all sides to work towards the goal. Physicians need to start their own "internal" reform, which essentially is to seek ways to make the services that they recommend and provide more cost-effective, and yet meet the needs of the patients that they serve. This would require a positive change in attitude toward healthcare ICT. How many physicians for example would doubt the value of evidence-based practice in rational care provision and resource optimization? From EMR (electronic medical record) to CPOE (computerized physician order entry), to RFID (Radio Frequency Identification), to a variety of DSS (decision support systems) available on the market, there are many other health ICT solutions that can enable physicians provide better quality and more cost-effective services. Physicians only need to embrace and adopt these technologies, albeit with some help from government and insurers, in the form of incentives and even financial support, which some countries already give. The public also needs reassurance, including that effective IT security are in place, regarding the safety and confidentiality of their personal information in order for them to feel more comfortable about electronic health/ medical records and to be more willing to participate in their use. Telehealth is making health services more accessible to persons living in remote and underserved areas, and electronic health record (EHR) is improving the quality of care by making crucial patient information available to physicians and other healthcare professionals in real time at the point of care (POC.) There is a lot more healthcare ICT is doing and can do to make the provision of qualitative, accessible, equitable, and sustainable health services what it should be in the new millennium. However, there is no gainsaying the need for concerted effort for these objectives to materialize.

The health systems of the UK, Canada, and the U.S have a number of differences, not least their funding systems, with a mix of public and private, essentially public, and private, funding systems, respectively. These different approaches to financing healthcare are in the main the reasons for the also significant differences in the organization and management of health services in these countries. However, and despite these differences, these health systems have a lot in common as well, including soaring healthcare costs that are guzzling significant portions of their GDP, on the one hand, yet proving incapable of meeting the ever-increasing healthcare needs of their peoples, with for example, millions in the U.S lacking health insurance, hence access to even minimal health services. Some of the healthcare reform models have reduced health spending in the past, for example in the U.S, some aspects of managed care, but as some would argue, at the expense of the consumer in particular whose ability to receive adequate healthcare, the activities of the non-medical administrators that determined the types and extent of services provided allegedly scandalously curtailed. The current focus in the U.S on consumer-driven healthcare is another attempt to reduce healthcare costs, predicated on the assumption that it would be the consumers' prerogative to choose preferred healthcare provider, but that they would be more discerning in making this choice and regarding their use of health services if they had to pay part of the costs. Another benefit expected of the model is the increased competition among providers that patients ability to choose providers would engender, competition that would modulate prices, eventually making healthcare more affordable, hence more accessible. In the event that this scenario worked, the ranks of the uninsured in the U.S would no doubt reduce. This indeed, is a desirable outcome, but there are important questions that need answers for it to materialize, the most crucial the consumer's ability to make rational choices. The consumer can only make rational choices, for example choosing an adept surgeon rather than a charlatan, armed with the necessary information to do so. Now, it is possible for the consumer to seek this information, but wherefrom? How could the consumer tell if a doctor was competent, incompetent, or has had, charges levied against him/ her for negligence? How would the consumer know if the price the provider offered him/ her for a procedure was competitive? How could we expect to realize the ideals of consumer-driven healthcare with the ability of healthcare consumers to make choices, the very core idea of the healthcare delivery model, compromised? What role could healthcare ICT play in providing consumers with the information that they need to make rational healthcare choices?

The publicly funded health system in Canada is also experiencing increasing healthcare costs. According to 2004 estimates, and at $31,500, Canada had the 12th highest GDP in the world, relative to the global average, which in U.S funds is $8,800, and to those of the U.S and the UK, $40,100, 2nd highest, and $29,600, 16th highest, respectively, on a purchasing power parity (PPP) basis and divided by population as of 1 July 2004. Despite spending an estimated over 10% of its GDP on healthcare in 2004, future spending projected to be even more, the country has a significant hospital wait list problems that has many clamoring for a parallel private health system to rectify this and other problems its health system faces that are unsatisfactory to many Canadians. There is no doubt that the wait list problem has a multi-faceted origin, but what role could healthcare ICT play in easing it, making healthcare more accessible to the people? Is it indeed, necessary to have a parallel private health system in Canada to solve its healthcare delivery problems, or is movement in this direction in fact inevitable? The 2005 Supreme Court ruling essentially allowing Quebecois to seek private health services if they did not want to be on hospital wait list has brought the private versus public health debate in the country forcefully to the fore. There is uncertainty about the ultimate outcome of this debate although some provinces even besides Quebec, for examples Alberta and British Columbia seem headed toward a parallel private health system? Could more widespread adoption of healthcare ICT by improving the processes involved in service delivery in the public health system avert this tendency? Is what the U.K health system also needs is a determined commitment toward healthcare ICT diffusion in order to solve its own equally pervasive hospital wait list problems? There is no doubt about the improvement in health service provision that automation brings, and this is irrespective of the health reform or funding model. This is because healthcare delivery is a conglomeration of processes, and funding or reform models do not determine or indeed rectify faulty processes, or could they not improve simply on account of these models? Indeed, the theme of this book is the need for appreciation of this process model of healthcare delivery as key to the way forward to solving the variety of problems health systems, including those of the countries analyzed in this book, confront. In fact, such an appreciation would make it easier to tackle the problems they would continue to confront as new challenges emerge due to the inevitable changes that come with time.

UK Health System in Transition

Arguably, the underlying philosophy of the U.K's National Health Service (NHS) needs overhauling. Taxpayer funded since found in 1947, some would insist that no alternative funding scheme would serve the country better. Others would point to its miscalculation of the power of consumer demand that the development of the services has coped well with rising consumer expectations of service provision over the years, particularly with no price deterrence operational, and no competitor with which to contend. Both positions were controversial, held tenaciously to by adherents. Even successive governments could least afford to change the health system but incrementally. Margaret Thatcher for example in 1990 retained public funding of the NHS but introduced some internal market reforms. Having purchasers and providers, the former essentially buying services from providers in the NHS assumed to be of better value than from other providers was indicative of the increasing recognition of the need for market forces to prevail even within the health industry, as "Hospital Trusts," with their budgets and goals, compete for purchasers' patronage. Disbursement of taxpayers' funds was at last seemingly cost-effective. Purchasing managers, hence patients, had choices, and providers, had to improve the quality of their services, or risk losing clientele. Enabling family doctors, or general practitioners, to form group practices and become "budget holders," equipped with the funds to provide their patients' total health services needs, including family care, specialist care, and hospital bills, also made them purchasers, albeit auxiliary, buying health services for patients in the internal market just as did the purchasing managers. NHS-employed, GPs were more venturesome, quality, and competition-driven, in purchasing services for their patients sometimes even offering novel value propositions to save costs buying similar services more exorbitantly, their wait times, reportedly falling well under the national average. Many more GPs later opted in, more than 50% of patients at one point with budget-holding practices. If the Internal market worked so well, why did the next government in 1997, a labor government "reform" it? Did it become top-heavy, with more managers than doctors required for healthcare delivery? Did bureaucracy, and complicated accounting and contractual systems stifle the reforms? Was market information to facilitate the mechanics of market forces lacking? How were the purchasers evaluating quality? Was it objective? Did the fact that some purchasers, perhaps flustered by the lack of benchmarks for comparative quality appraisal resort to block-contract negotiating, for all procedures and services in order to receive budget pricing compromise market operations, and eventually the NHS? Could these problems have informed the decision of this labor government to set up new purchasing organizations, with the involvement of an array of health professionals and not just family doctors? How could more-effective deployment of information technologies have helped Thatcherian internal market reforms work better? Some contend that the new arrangement is merely an extension of the former, and perhaps one fraught with problems from the start, hence moribund just like its predecessor, its more centralized nature antithetical to the competitive underpinning of market forces, and would the novel idea of "earned autonomy" the government proposes to give NHS units of proven quality the answer? Is it a reversal to the concept of a decentralized provider sector? In what direction could healthcare information and communications technologies (ICT) have influenced these developments, and in which, is it doing so now? Could health information technologies be the underlying common strand that binds the answers to the variety of problems that the UK NHS currently confronts? Much has occurred in the UK healthcare scene in the intervening years. Commissions on health services have submitted reports. Policy changes have prevailed over their antecedents, and others have receded into oblivion. Parliamentary debates have raged, for example recently, over policy details on not whether there is anything wrong with a particular antismoking legislation, but on circumstances fit for exemption. Wait times continue to feature prominently, some would argue perhaps pre-eminently, in health policy decisions. The changes to the health system seem to continue ad infinitum, but are these because something is missing that is critical to finding the definitive answers to the country's healthcare problems, or is it inevitable that healthcare, just as everything else in life, is subject to change? Even if this were so, is it also inevitable that change be painful? Could changes in the health system not be methodical, predicated upon anticipated, if not even planned transition? Should we, for example, not expect the system to require certain changes based on known and estimated health statistics such as infant mortality rates? Could we also not control what to expect in the final analysis? Could we not for example, control disease prevalence hence have an accurate idea of future prevalence hence health needs regarding the disease, and in turn, resource allocation? If indeed, it is possible to achieve these objectives, would it not put us more in control of health spending? How much could we save having such control, and could the effect of such control not trickle down, at the very least to spending in other services, for example, social services? Would society in general not be moving closer to rational resource allocation that would ensure fiscal balance, hence sustainable development? These questions suggest that healthcare delivery plays a central role in the overall affairs of any society. However, healthcare delivery could not, on its own achieve the goals that the questions raised above aim to achieve. A variety of factors for example, progress in medical knowledge, drug research, and technological innovation, availability and distribution of healthcare professionals, public policy changes, emerging diseases, and even health and other issues in other parts of the world, could be crucial to the success or otherwise of healthcare delivery. Of all these various factors however, innovations in healthcare ICT promises to provide the UK health system the veritable cobblestones that would pave the path of future progress. Consider recent advances in the study of sleep for example. Some people have problems falling asleep, some wake up too early, in other words, do not sleep long enough, yet others have interrupted, non-restorative sleep, and some just cannot keep their eyes open, or put differently, cannot stay awake. These are only a few of the known sleep-wakefulness disorders, although there are many more, and they affect people young and old, male and female, about 20% of the population suffering from one or another sleep disorder, not to mention the associated psychological burden of sleep deprivation, and the consequent depression and anxiety related diseases in some patients. Sleep disorders are some of the commonest disorders that children have for example, with infant sleep rhythm complaints by new mothers up to 46%, the prevalence of childhood obstructive sleep apnea, 2%, adolescent problems even more prevalent. Indeed, there are over 80 (International Classification of Diseases) ICD-9 classified sleep disorders, their causes, clinical presentation, treatment, and outcomes, just as varied, for example the masking of the symptoms of narcolepsy until past adolescence, hence easy for doctors to sometimes miss the diagnosis of this and other sleep disorders, with attendant consequences for the patient and for service utilization[1].

Misdiagnosis indeed is itself of increasing concern and was number one on a list of medical mistakes that patients say they have experienced, according to a recent online survey of over 2,000 U.S. respondents that a UK marketing firm YouGov, conducted. The survey asked people in the United States if in the past five years, they had experienced or knew somebody who had experienced a medical error, to which about a third of the participants responded affirmatively, and the rest, negatively. Fifty percent of those who had experienced a medical mistake attributed it to misdiagnosis or diagnostic delay, 24 percent or someone they knew, to medication error, and 18 percent, to an error made during an operation or procedure. Commissioned by the U.K. firm, Isabel Healthcare, which makes decision-support (DSS) software that enables doctors to enter free-text regarding a patient's symptoms, and then match these with possible diagnoses, an almost tragic personal experience due to a misdiagnosis of a potentially-life threatening flesh-eating disease for chicken pox in a UK hospital inspired the survey. It also did, the software to assist diagnosis, and ensure patient safety, an example of the interplay of factors mentioned earlier that could influence the direction of healthcare delivery[2]. In particular, it exemplifies the role that healthcare ICT could play as an underlying but unifying force in the ever-unfolding dynamics of the array of factors on which this direction depends. Paradoxically, it also typifies the slow pace of adoption in the health industry of these technologies, despite their evident potential to improve healthcare delivery and simultaneously save costs. Only a few healthcare organizations have adopted this valuable software, for example, Loma Linda University School of Medicine and Children's Hospital adopted it, its U.S. market penetration estimated at less than 2%. Could this be due to minimal interest in the issue of misdiagnosis as a patient safety issue, and why, especially with the Institute of Medicine (IOM) report only five years ago that showed close to ninety nine thousand people die in the US annually due to medical errors? Is misdiagnosis not a medical error, and could it not jeopardize patient safety as with the misdiagnosis of a potentially fatal illness for chicken pox mentioned above? According Dr. William Munier, acting director of the Agency for Healthcare Research and Quality's Center for Quality Improvement "Disease is complex, patients are complex," adding that the medical community is not disinterested in misdiagnosis, but that it is more difficult to quantify without adequate data, or even obtain a consensus on among healthcare professionals. For example, amputating the right rather than the left leg, an error of commission, would receive probably attention, but not a misdiagnosis, an error of omission. However, could such an error of omission in a misdiagnosis of acute appendicitis not lead to peritonitis and possibly death? Should an error of commission, such as an elective plantar wart excision instead of a forehead lipoma, warrant an internal inquiry? Munier and a senior fellow at the Institute for Healthcare Improvement and senior consultant Dana-Farber Cancer Institute, Jim Conway, envision information technologies playing a role in changing things. According to Conway, "One of the powerful things that the computer brings is the way it presents information," adding "The whole role of the electronic medical record and how it brings together information can reduce misdiagnosis and delayed diagnosis." Munier agrees but adds that measuring quality outcomes in healthcare will have to improve in tandem with the evolution of electronic medical records (EMR). Emerging healthcare ICT aimed at helping prevent the misdiagnosis of sleep disorders illustrate these points. Among adults, insomnia, the subjective complaint of inadequate sleep quantity or quality, is the commonest sleep disorder, followed by excessive daytime somnolence, which latter may itself be due to insomnia, and causes significant morbidity and mortality, including about 200,000 automobile crashes occur annually due to drivers excessive sleepiness[2]. There is even some link between daytime somnolence and major disasters for example the mistaken launch of the Challenger space shuttle (1986), and it impairs learning and cognitive processes[3]. Expensive and complicated diagnostic and management limited how much help patients received for their sleep problems, but that is about to change, with a novel approach researchers have recently developed to measure sleep, the IST project SENSATION[4]. The project comprises 46 partners from 20 different countries. The goal of SENSATION is to explore a variety of micro- and nano-sensor technologies, in order to achieve "unobtrusive, cost-effective, real-time monitoring, detection and prediction of human physiological state in relation to wakefulness, fatigue and stress anytime, everywhere and for everybody"[4]. The scientists aim to develop a multipurpose sensing platform comprising 17 micro sensors and 2 nano sensors, linked via a local area network (LAN). They will analyze the different states of human brain within Subproject 1, and develop

17 micro sensors and two nano sensors in Subproject 2, including wearable, eye-related posture and motility and autonomic functions sensors that will monitor brain activity, and they will integrate all the sensors wirelessly via a body/ local/ wide area network. They will integrate the sensors with medical systems for medical diagnosis and treatment in Subproject 3, and with a system for operator's hypovigilance detection and prediction, for industrial use in Subproject 4, and in Subproject 5, coordinate the overall IP via a number of cross-project activities. The sensors will make it unnecessary for example to spend nights in a sleep lab for sleep-studies measurements since your sensor-laden mattress at home would enable taking the measurements at home, making these studies more convenient, cheaper, even more reliable. According to Dr Evangelos Bekiaris of the Greece Centre for Research & Technology Hellas / Hellenic Institute of Transport, it is possible to integrate the sensors into other things, namely, bed and pillow textiles, wrist straps, seat linings, even the frames of reading glasses. The sensors are able to measure brain activity, heart rate, and eye and muscle movements via wireless integration with a computer network, while an individual is awake or asleep, the data collected in a body area network, transmitted wirelessly to a LAN, and then to the hospital for analysis. Applications of the sensors include safe monitoring and early warning of individuals as they conduct their daily routines, for examples those operating critical machinery such as anesthetic equipments, nuclear reactors, or air traffic controllers, or driving vehicles, for example, on a long haul, preventing them falling asleep, as sleeping under such circumstances could have catastrophic consequences. Statistics show an association between 25% of the traffic accidents in the UK, or 40 per cent in the US, and driver fatigue. The scientists estimate that by alerting people before and not after they fall asleep as current devices are only able to do, the SENSATION sleep platform with its sensors could reduce serious road accidents by 30%, and industrial accidents by more than 15%. Other application areas include monitoring aircraft pilots to ensure they do not fall asleep, babies to prevent cot death, or to manage sleep, for example appraise one's sleep pattern hence plan shift work based on the determined biorhythms. Does this technology not offer enhanced features for sleep studies and create precise data gathering, analysis, and utilization, including for accurate diagnosis and the institution of appropriate measures whose outcomes are measurable? Does it not point in the direction of the future of sleep management in

health and in disease, offer options for reducing morbidities and mortalities related to sleep deprivation? Does it not offer opportunities for intersectoral collaboration on policy formulation and for optimization of resource allocation and utilization, hence for reducing overall healthcare costs? Does it also not provide opportunities for technological deployment that could promote competition among healthcare providers, facilitate the efficient operations of the healthcare markets, and create opportunities for patient empowerment, including choice of provider? Could seeking answers to these questions, those posed earlier, and similar questions not be one likely effective approach to envisioning healthcare delivery in the UK in the years ahead? Would such an approach not provide the most inclusive solutions to even some of the seemingly most intractable problems confronting the country s health system, for example the hospital wait-list problem?

A new Temple University study published in the March 2006 issue of the Journal of Health Communication illustrates these points. The study notes that newly diagnosed cancer patients that use the Internet to seek information on their disease have a more positive outlook, and some even participated more actively in their treatments. As trivial as this may seem to some, this pioneer study of the relationship between Internet use and patient behaviors, speaks for the increasing interest of patients and individuals in general in information on wellness, illnesses, and other health issues. It also confirms that access to readily available health information could help increase treatment compliance and patients to cope with treatment side effects and other issues related to their illnesses. The researchers recruited patients who called a U.S. National Cancer Institute-funded 1-800 number. Trained specialists answered questions about the disease and directed callers to cancer-related resources in their area. There were 442 participants classified into "direct user, indirect user and non user" categories based on their Internet usage patterns, with direct and indirect users mostly females, 50 to 60 years old, were college graduates, and earned over $60,000 a year. The researchers observed notable links between Internet use and the patients' feelings about their treatment, with those that used the Internet and that received Internet information from family members or friends likelier to view their relationship with their doctors as a partnership, and were more comfortable to ask questions and challenge treatment alternatives. According to the principal investigator and public health Professor Sarah Bass, PhD, "They saw the Internet as a powerful tool that enhanced their decision-making ability". The researchers also observed that many early non-users after eight weeks turned to the Internet for information, about 75% of these attributing the change on questioning to encouragement by either family/ friend or to the cancer diagnosis itself prompting them to increase their Internet use. "They didn't want to feel powerless or have to rely on the doctor to make all of the decisions," said Professor Bass, who noted that now is the time for doctors and health workers to encourage patients to do their own research on the Web, with the increasing slash in funding for medical phone hotlines. The professor also noted, "But as with most things, let the buyer beware. Stick to Web sites that are associated with large, well-recognized non-profit groups, or get recommendations from your physician." Should health systems, including in the UK not capitalize on this thirst for health information, which is not restricted to the U.S but rather is an expression of a universal human attribute to enquire? Has this exploratory tendency not been the underlying driving force for the successes of humankind we all enjoy today, including the emergence of the Internet itself, in which it only now seeks fulfillment? Should we then extinguish this innate tendency now or nurture it even more vigorously in an age that even tiny microbes that we need high-resolution microscopes to see threaten to wipe us off the face of the earth with insidious pandemics, and soaring health spending, nations with economic collapse? To think that it is possible to prevent and stop these microbes and health spending in the main makes the thought of extinguishing the quest for information by the public unthinkable. On the contrary, is this not an age that people should have even more health information that could help with health promotion, and disease prevention? Does the above study not provide evidence of the key role that the Internet could play in providing such information? In fact, the Internet is only one of the many ways healthcare ICT could help provide individuals with health information. Some might cringe at the idea of providing people with more information considering what they would term the "information overload" already present. True, a cursory surfing of the Internet for example would reveal many Web sites purporting to give health information, but a significant number of these Web sites only provide inaccurate and stale information, and even worse often slanted to meet the marketing needs of these Web sites, which was probably why Professor Bass issued the cautionary statement quoted above. Few would disagree that this is not the sort of health information that the public needs, and that if anything, such information actually puts people's lives in danger. On the other hand, we need to avoid an information glut even providing individuals with current, accurate, timely, and unbiased health information, which is why the concept of targeted health information provision becomes crucial, and underscores the increasing need for the deployment of relevant healthcare ICT, which could play a vital role in achieving this goal. With important new knowledge on health and disease targeted at those that need them in a timely manner, there is no gainsaying the benefits this would afford people in preventing illnesses, living a healthy life, knowing all they need to know about their ailments, and improving their quality of life (QOL). Would these benefits not also reduce health services utilization, particularly hospitalization rates and stays hence hospital wait lists and prescription drugs costs? Should the U.K health system not be exploring the technologies that could enable such targeted health information and the approaches to deploying them in order to achieve this objective of health information going to the people that need them, who then have the option to avoid getting lost in the health information maze out there on the Internet and elsewhere? Should we not be increasingly employing novel, "out-of-the box" approaches to solving contemporary healthcare delivery problems in the U.K. exploring the immense opportunities health information technologies offer us in so doing? Critics of national health care systems such as the NHS insist that such systems typically ration healthcare delivery, for examples by not covering certain types of treatment, or by imposing cost constraints via budgets, or limited technology, even wait times. Some estimates suggest that a million people in the UK await admission to NHS hospitals at any point in time, with 100,000 cancellations of surgical procedures annually. Canada also confronts troubling wait times problems, and in New Zealand, about 90,000 await surgery per year, and Sweden has up to a 25-week, wait time for heart surgery$_6$. The question then arises, if these figures should remain the way they are and if they should not, how to bring them down. Is not bringing the figures down not going to mean continued escalation of health spending, which would likely be increasingly difficult to finance? Some argue that even in countries such as Canada with its budget surpluses in recent years is only able to support the rising health spending because the provinces are receiving Federal largesse that these surpluses fund, which begs the question regarding where the funds would come from if the budget surplus ceased. In any case, it is fiscally prudent to contain costs, be they in healthcare or other services, but should such cost containment compromise health service delivery? Is it not possible to contain costs while simultaneously delivering qualitative, comprehensive, accessible, and affordable health services? Some contend that one of the major problems with the U.S. health system is that the people spending the country's health money are not the ones paying the bills, with attendant misuse/ abuse of the health systems, which is one reason they call for cost sharing. The idea is that this would make healthcare consumers more discerning in their use of health services, but would consumers not need reliable and accurate information about the prices of procedures, and other healthcare products and services, their quality and safety, and on healthcare professionals for them to make rational choices? Would such information not make it easier for them to choose the best quality services at the most affordable prices? Would such decisions not compel healthcare providers to improve their services and not to price themselves out of the market? Is it not again clear that healthcare ICT has a key underlying role in the actualization of these processes? Would providing U.K healthcare consumers with the necessary information not facilitate the sort of consumer empowerment described above? Would it not make for a more effective and responsive market that consumers, and insurers and employers control the money? The point here is that even in a publicly funded health system there is a limit beyond which rising healthcare costs should not go in the interest of the overall economy of the country. Yet, we cannot wish the increasing demand for better health service provision by the public away. No one would say for example that it is wrong for the public to demand a reduction in hospital wait times. This means that it is imperative to seek ways to meet public expectation of health service provision without the economy having to collapse. It is therefore unlikely that any healthcare stakeholder s disinterest in what healthcare ICT could help achieve in this regard belies an appreciation of the evidently immense benefits derivable from healthcare ICT adoption. This is why a significant part of the efforts to promote healthcare ICT diffusion in Britain and in any country for that matter involves changing end-user attitudes. This in turn calls for understanding the underlying issues that hinder and would encourage healthcare professionals in particular to embrace and implement healthcare ICT.

To underscore the need for such efforts, consider the findings in a recent study on medication errors[7]. Medication errors in the intensive care unit (ICU) are common and result in patient morbidity and mortality, increased length of ICU stay and considerable added costs. The researchers sought to know if the introduction of a computerized ICU system (Centricity Critical Care Clinisoft, GE Healthcare) reduced the incidence and severity of medication prescription errors (MPEs). They conducted a prospective trial in a paper-based unit (PB-U) versus a computerized unit (C-U) in a 22-bed ICU of a tertiary university hospital, all medication order and medication prescription error validated by a clinical pharmacist, the severity of MPEs evaluated by a neutral panel. The researchers split MPEs into three groups, namely, minor MPEs, with no potential to cause harm; intercepted MPEs, with the potential to cause harm but intercepted on time; and serious MPEs, which were non-intercepted potential adverse drug events (ADE) or ADEs, that is, MPEs with potential to cause, or actually causing, patient harm. The C-U and the PB-U each had 80 patient-days, medication prescriptions assessed were 2,510, MPEs identified, 375, their incidence significantly lower in the C-U compared with the PBU (3.4%) versus (27.0%). The researchers also found significantly less minor MPEs in the C-U than in the PB-U, and lower intercepted MPEs in the C-U and the non-intercepted potential ADEs, which were also lower in the C-U, although they found no fatal errors. The authors also found that the most frequent drug classes involved were cardiovascular medication and antibiotics in both groups, and that patients who had kidney failure experienced less dosing errors in the C-U, and concluded that the ICU computerization, including the medication order entry, led to a significant decrease in the incidence and severity of medication errors in the ICU. Numerous other studies have demonstrated the value of CPOE, and other healthcare ICT, and the varieties of new technologies introduced at the ongoing CeBit 2006 (March 9-15, 2006) in Hannover, Germany attests to the wide range of opportunities that the health industry has in applying these technologies to improve healthcare delivery. The dominant themes at the fair are convergence and mobility, essentially the convergence of a number of different technologies into one versatile, portable device creating immense options for consumers for multimodal experience on the go. Microsoft's mini PC project Origami, which the Korean electronics firm Samsung calls Q1, and plans to start selling in just another few weeks, a paperback sized ultra-portable, computer with a 7-inch touchscreen, a 40 gigabyte hard drive, an Intel Celeron processor, runs the tablet edition of Windows XP, and uses Wi-Fi, and Bluetooth to communicate, is one such device. This device, which has extra features, for example a Bluetooth keyboard and a card that enables it to communicate using mobile phone networks, is sure to be one that doctors in the U.K and elsewhere would likely embrace, being so portable, weighing only 779g, and could easily fit into the pocket of their white clinic coats. There is no doubt that it would facilitate not just communication between doctors and their patients but also with other healthcare professionals and access to patient information at the point of care (POC), enhancing patient safety. Because this device could perform all the tasks that a regular PC does, and runs in two modes, as a chopped down PC running the familiar Windows operating system (OS), and as simply a media device, enabling users watch video or listen to music without turning on the OS, it promises to be a valuable resource for targeted information sharing. Individuals could access such information in a variety of multimedia formats in real time or download, store and later, access it, at their convenience. Indeed, Samsung s device also has a Digital Media Broadcasting tuner that enables it to handle TV programs broadcast for mobile gadgets. The increasing convergence in the computer industry bodes well for improved healthcare delivery with consumers having a single mobile computing device that offers the mobile functionality of many diverse devices. According to Samsung, the Q1 billed to cost £ 699 (1,000 euros) would replace mobile media players, game handhelds, palmtop computers, and notebook PCs. Asustek, the Chinese Founder Group, and Intel are all working on their own designs for the ultra-portable PC, and other portable devices were also on display at the fair, for example mobile phones with live TV features. Is it not worth trying to promote the adoption of these technologies by the people that need to use them for the health system to enjoy these benefits? It is of course unlikely that we would cover all the small details of the efforts required to make the impact of healthcare ICT felt, but suffice to point in the general direction of the strategic shift necessary to achieve this goal. One of the key issues discussed thus far, that of targeted information provision via appropriate information technologies is at the very core of the shift in focus of healthcare delivery in the U.K. that could provide the synthesis of its underlying social value with the imperative the continuing shifts in orientation in the healthcare arena and technological progress command. In other words, that the country needs to focus on disease prevention, health promotion, and public health, and on efforts to ensure tighter integration of health and social services, among other intersectoral collaborative initiatives, is not just fiscally prudent, but also in keeping with the renewed vigor such efforts deserve in an increasingly intercalated world. Is it any wonder that the head of the World Trade Organization (WTO) said on Wednesday March 08, 2006, that health takes priority over international trade agreements and intellectual property as the world tries to fight the threat of bird flu, which had infected 175 people and killed 96 of them since 2003? "To the question of whether a WTO member can put up obstacles to trade as a consequence of a threat to public health, the answer is yes, .each member has room to move if there is a threat. It is not unlimited (room) under the system, but health trumps trade if necessary," WTO Director-General Pascal Lamy told a business meeting in Madrid. The World Health Organization (WHO) had earlier urged people to take action in preparation for a widespread outbreak of bird flu, to develop vaccines, stockpile medicines, and educate people. Do these statements not buttress the point about the need for efforts aimed at disease prevention? Should the U.K wait for an outbreak of bird flu before taking action, for example? Are the measures these world leaders suggested also not indicative of a major role for healthcare ICT in such preventive efforts? Could healthcare ICT not help in preventing other diseases? Although the WTO boss did not specify the rules, he made clear that regarding producing medicines and antivirals, a public health emergency would trump intellectual property rules the organization, which in the past allowed members to waive patents on medicines to combat specific health challenges, had set. Now that animals, for example cats, other than birds have bird flu, how much longer would it take for human-to-human transmission of the virus to occur? Indeed, is an avian flue pandemic in the horizon, and if so, when would it happen? Could we still do something to prevent this doomsday scenario? This human-to-human transmission does not have to start in the UK. How long does it take an infected individual in any other country, who might not even realize he/ she has the infection, before embarking on a vacation, or business trip to London arrive there? Again, is it any wonder that the United States, Switzerland and Singapore have proposed that countries eliminate tariffs on medicines and medical devices as part of a new world trade deal, according to U.S. trade officials in a statement on Monday, February 27, 2006s? The United Nations estimated almost $33 billion in yearly pharmaceutical trade and $23 billion in medical equipment trade are subject to import duties, more often than not by developing countries, and as the U.S. Trade Representative s office noted, the very countries in urgent need of cheap medicines. Would lifting these tariffs combined with developed countries in which most of the major drug companies are not seeking drug patent protections in trade pacts that invariably also increase the cost of medicines in these developing countries, not help the preventive and curative efforts in the latter countries? Indeed, a recent joint research paper from the American Enterprise Institute and the Brookings Institution concluded that elimination of tariffs and taxes on essential drugs would likely save thousands of lives across the developing world." Could this prevention in one country of a disease not prevent its emergence in another? These examples illustrate the increasing importance of disease prevention and the need for not only in country, intersectoral but also cross-country collaboration in achieving this goal. In other words, the UK health system needs to be looking both inward and outward in conceptualizing its approaches to healthcare delivery in the years ahead and information technologies are crucial tools in these efforts. It is no doubt top priority for the government to seek ways to prevent diseases in the country but it should also contribute to global efforts in preventing diseases in general, which would no doubt be in the interest of the U.K ultimately. Is it therefore surprising that the United Kingdom, the Netherlands, and Ireland on Tuesday March 07, 2006, announced donations totaling about $14.2 million to the Global Alliance for TB Drug Development for the development of new tuberculosis treatments, according to Reuters South Africa? The U.K. plans to provide about $11.4 million, the Netherlands, about $2.4 million, and Ireland, about $357,000 over three years. Approaches to health reforms would increasingly be broader based, encompassing issues both internal and external to the country, and not necessarily only those in the health domain. Would knowledge of customs and practices of immigrants for example, including estimates of their numbers over time not be sine qua non for effective present and future health-policy formulation? How would the increasing mobility of individuals, for work, holidays, and other purposes, particularly with U.K being in the ever-enlarging European Union (EU) determine telecommunications legislation and health policies? Would it not be desirable for a U.K resident or an Emergency room (ER) doctor looking after him/ her to have ready access to his/ her health records if he/ she took ill suddenly while vacationing in Brussels, for example? Does this not support the need for nationwide health information network and widespread adoption of electronic health records (EHR) systems? Does it in fact not suggest the need to develop the necessary information technologies, and regulatory polices, for cross-border collaboration for health information communication and sharing? The Global Alliance is developing 10 compounds and is testing Bayer's drug moxifloxacin, in the hope that by 2010, the addition of moxifloxacin to a novel TB treatment would reduce treatment time from six to between two and three months. Is it not important to target this information at those that need it? Targeting health information to the right persons not only facilitates disease prevention and health promotion, it is also an integral aspect of the treatment of diseases, and technology-enabled, evidence-based medicine is proving to be an asset in this regard. For example, Dr. Carolyn Clancy, Director of the US Agency for Healthcare Research and Quality (AHRQ) recently introduced the agency s Effective Health Care Program a new software program that enables doctors and their patients to compare treatments for high-priority medical disorders, in order to see which ones has evidence to show that it is the most effective[9]. This evidence-based medicine program has already produced its first comparative effectiveness report on treatment alternatives for gastric reflux disease, the agency planning to release reports on breast cancer diagnosis, arthritis, heart disease, Alzheimer s, and other important topics in 2006. One of the issues the agency is looking into is how best to disseminate these reports so that more practitioners, purchasers, and consumers can use the information. This again emphasizes the need for targeted information dissemination in healthcare, which existing information technologies for examples, the Internet, e-mails, text messaging, mobile phones, some with live TV features lately, VoIP, BlackBerrys, Palm Pilots, or Pocket PCs, and others could help with. Emerging technologies, such as those that enable computer analyses of structured and unstructured information, including integrating and analyzing the combined data offer immense opportunities for such information transmission too. How much could we achieve by targeting important health information at young people, for example regarding the dangers of substance abuse, teenage pregnancies, recklessness, and crime. Could a youngster who engaged in arson that he/ she called a prank and a mistake have learnt not do so via targeted information, or could a teenager who thinks it is "cool" to smoke cigarettes because his peers are doing so? Could we be nurturing a new generation of healthy adults whose exposure to vital health information at an early age led to avoidance of unhealthy lifestyles? Much is made of the aging population of many Western countries regarding the likely increase in health spending taking care of their healthcare needs would entail, but a recent US census report suggests that the effect of aging baby boomer population might be less than predicted in part because of fewer elderly people with disabilities. The report, which the US Census Bureau released on Thursday March 09, 2006, indicates that older U.S. residents are living longer, healthier lives with fewer disabilities[10]. Titled, "65+ in the United States: 2005," researchers from the Census Bureau and the National Institute on Aging collated population data from Census surveys and other federal sources, for example the CDC, the Bureau of Labor Statistics, and Medicare claims, for the study. The researchers noted that the proportion of individuals over age 65 who had a disability described in the report as "a substantial limitation in major life activity" fell from 26.2% in 1982 to 19.7% in 1999, a pattern expected to continue, higher education levels thought in part responsible for the improved health. This again underlines the importance of health information, and in particular, the added advantages of such information targeted contextually at the right people at the right time, and in the most appropriate mode. It also highlights the future benefits on health of targeting health information earlier on in life. Furthermore, consider the researchers estimates of the increase in the US population of persons over age 65 to 72 million by 2030 from about 36 million in 2000, and of those above 85 years to double to 9.6 million during the same time period. Consider also that almost one in five U.S. residents to be 65 or older by 2030, compared with 12% presently, what would the picture be like on health spending were theses seniors not highly informed including about their health? How would it look for the future of healthcare delivery in the U.K that there is minimal curative and more preventive health service utilization in future? Would the population not be healthier, and would healthcare spending not be much less, freeing resources for use in other areas? Would it be difficult to engage young people, who are literally growing up in an information technology age, with important health information targeted at them via their iPods, increasingly sophisticated cell phones, PlayStations and X-boxes, or via pop vending machines, and movies both at home and in theaters? One important requirement for acceptance of such information, of course would be for it to be contextual in many ways, the language, the media, the timing, the amount, and the like, attributes of the targeted information, incidentally applicable to different target groups, and which appropriate experts could help put together, again with the aid of sophisticated computer algorithms, for example. Would young people not relate better for example with an anti-smoking campaign that emphasizes that it is "uncool" to smoke and expect a peck or a kiss than a bunch of gross pictures of smoking-related diseases on cigarette packs? Health information targeted at the appropriate population could significantly help prevention efforts, at all levels, and not only with disease prevention, which is the primary level. Knowing the symptoms and signs of a disease could increase the index of suspicion of an individual and prompt the person to seek medical help. Would it not help an individual at high risk for a certain health problem, for example, diabetes, known to be relatively common among blacks and Hispanics, and in overweight and obese persons, for examples, to know its clinical presentation, particularly as type-2 diabetes could be latent in such individuals for many years, damaging their organs surreptitiously? What would such persons, or those that know someone who is prone to or has the condition, subscribing to targeted health information a health information firm, government health information unit, physician practices with comprehensive value proposition, or healthcare advocacy groups with dedicated health information portals, for examples, lose? With obesity rates among U.S seniors, increasing for example, and about 33% of senior men and 39% of senior women obese does this not suggest, the need for targeted health information to be ongoing considering the benefits to their health mentioned earlier of U.S seniors being highly educated? Would these benefits, including on the likelihood of lesser health spending not vanish if the seniors did not continue to receive health information, which in any case has the propensity to change with advances in medical knowledge as the following example shows? The European Prospective Investigation into Cancer and Nutrition (EPIC) study reported in September 2003 that one could reduce the risk of colorectal cancer, in particular of the left colon, by 40% by simply doubling the low average intake of dietary fiber[11]. Even at the time, the results contradicted those of many other studies, although with half a million participants, aged 27 to 70 years, spread over ten European countries, they were difficult to dismiss. However, recent data from thirteen prospective cohort trials of 725,628 men and women also run counter to the EPIC trial[12], despite a similar range of fiber intake. These recent data showed negligible risk reduction, although fruit and cereal fiber showed non-significant protection in age-adjusted model, after multiple adjustments. Vegetables, on the other hand, showed no effect whatsoever. Research evidence also indicates that fiber seems ineffective in protecting against colonic polyp recurrence, often considered the surrogate marker for colon cancer, studies criticized for the cereal fiber being wheat fiber, and not mixed cereals such as oats and barley, and the fruit and vegetable intake being low at lower than five servings a day. Other researchers argue that may be dietary fiber intake of over 10g/ day would protect against colorectal cancer, which they conceptualized as a 'fiber deficiency disease'. Considering that average fiber intake among Ugandans, is well over 70g/ day, which is very high relative to those in these studies, observations in whom led Denis Burkitt to first propose this hypothesis, may provide some insight into the current controversy. Nonetheless, it is important to remember that there is none over the benefits of fiber in reducing the risk of coronary heart disease (CHD). Would it not be necessary to provide individuals at risk for colorectal cancer, and heart diseases, such important information as above, indeed, the data and information analyzed and presented in the most appropriate form that would ensure their receipt, and understanding? What would software and ICT vendors in the U.K or elsewhere lose developing the required tools and programs to provide such services?

Diabetes is becoming more prevalent in the U.K. In 2004, about 1.8 million persons in the country had the disease, about 250,000 people, Type 1 diabetes, and a little over 1.5 million, Type 2 diabetes, according to the charity, Diabetes UK, an increase of 400,000 in only eight years, 3% of the total population, a continuing increase expected as the population ages and becomes more overweight. Two years ago, the NHS spent about £ 10m a day, or 5% of its budget, on treating diabetes and its complications, this percentage expected to increase to 10% by 2011. Would preventing diabetes, primary prevention, not be a worthwhile goal, or its early diagnosis and treatment, secondary prevention, with estimates of those at the time that had latent, undiagnosed Type 2 diabetes at up to a million? Would these not reduce the strain on local NHS services to establish the required services to minimize its sequelae, a process termed tertiary prevention? Could targeted health information not help in achieving all of these prevention goals? Controlling diabetes effectively could reduce the risk of heart disease by 44%, that of stroke by 46%, eye and kidney diseases by 33% each. Controlling Type 1 diabetes effectively could cut the risk of developing new eye disease by as much as 76%, and of existing ones becoming worse by 54%. It could reduce the risk of nerve damage by 60%, of developing kidney disease, and of existing kidney disease becoming worse by 54% and 39%, respectively. Are the benefits of secondary prevention of diabetes not therefore immediately obvious, benefits derivable by the delivery of healthcare ICT-enabled targeted health information to those persons that really need them? As Dr Graham Archard, the then Royal College of General Practitioners (RCGP) spokesperson said, "It is clear that diabetes and the related problem of obesity is now a major health concern in the UK and it looks like its only going to get worse before it gets better." With Type 1 reducing life expectancy by two decades on the average and Type 2 diabetes by one, half of individuals diagnosed with the latter already suffering complications of the disease by the time they receive the diagnosis, there is little doubt about the need for preventing the disease, and treating it promptly and effectively. Diabetes is the number one cause of blindness among working people in the U.K where individuals with the disease spend 1.1 million days each year in hospital, are thrice more likely have a stroke than those that do not have the disease, and 80% die from its cardiovascular complications. U.K's National Diabetes Support Team (NDST) is assisting to provide help and support to local services in implementing the National Service Framework for Diabetes (NSF,) with its Web site offering relevant information on the disease and individuals the opportunity to sign up for periodic Diabetes NSF briefing[13]. It also offers opportunities for effective information sharing and exchange. To be sure, the increasing prevalence of diabetes is not peculiar to the U.K. Indeed, 5% of the world's population has the condition and its prevalence is doubling every generation. About 200,000 people have diabetes in Ireland, Type-2 diabetes the commoner form, accounting for 85% of cases, with obesity and physical inactivity the main culprits[14]. The number of blind people in Ireland has increased by 37% in less than ten years, mainly due to diabetes, the prevalence of diabetic retinopathy (DR) increased by 120% from 147 to 323 people, including many young people. Recent studies in the U.K showed a similar pattern of increasing prevalence of diabetes among youths, who are also increasingly obese, the risk of developing Type 2 diabetes in obese individuals up 10 times, from 10 to 100 new cases annually. Researchers at the Royal College of Pediatrics and Child Health recently noted that increasing obesity rates have triggered a crisis of "adult" diabetes in children. The prevalence of Type 2 diabetes, which normally affects overweight people in middle age, increased 10-fold in the past five years, which experts described as "shocking". Worse still, the researchers, who conducted a national audit of all NHS diagnoses of Type 2 diabetes in under-16s in 2004-5, regard the 100-a-year figure as a likely pointer to a more prevalent problem because many parents may not appreciate that their gravely overweight children are presenting the early signs of diabetes. The experts also observed that another 60,000 children are suffering weight-related metabolic syndrome, which is a combination of conditions, namely high blood pressure, increased cholesterol and fats in the blood, among others, and which herald Type 2 diabetes. Why then, with all these staggering statistics and the activities of organizations such as NDST, most people who have a high risk of developing diabetes are unaware they are in danger of developing the condition, according to a survey by the charity, Diabetes UK published on March 01, 2006[16]? Does this not support the need for targeted health information, and that we should not wait for people to rummage through the World Wide Web, but should deliver the necessary and contextual information to them, via the appropriate healthcare ICT? Would the costs in organizing the delivery of such targeted information not pale in significance compared to the overall health benefits derivable from such an exercise, both in human and material terms? The U.K Department of Health plans the first anti-obesity public health campaign for later in 2006. Does this not offer a chance to implement this concept of information technology-enabled, targeted current, and relevant health information delivered to parents, youngsters, and others that need the information? The number of obese children increased from 9.6% in 1995 to 13.7% in 2003, the overall cost of obesity to the NHS, currently about £1bn/ annum, with additional £ 2.3bn to £ 2.6bn for the economy as a whole. More than 13% of children under 11 years old in England are obese, up from 9.6% in 1995, with the UK having one of the highest obesity rates in Europe, over thrice the French levels, although less the US and Mexico, for examples. Should the public not be looking to the government for leadership in establishing the required initiatives, including healthcare-ICT enabled targeted health education campaign aimed at tackling this increasingly troubling, what some called the "Diabetes Crisis"? As previously noted, is investing in tackling obesity in childhood and adolescence not deliberately nurturing a generation of healthier, fitter future adults? Would this not reduce morbidities and mortalities in future from obesity and related conditions, most of which actually become chronic, increasing hospital bed utilization, prescription drug costs, and overall healthcare spending? The government set the targets in July 2004 via intersectoral collaboration of the various partnerships between councils, the NHS, voluntary sector, and schools for tackling childhood obesity. Some criticize these as slow, as almost two years into the campaign key parts of the delivery plan remain unpublished and guidance to primary care trusts on measuring children only published in January 2006, hence, measurement of young people will unlikely commence until the summer, preliminary results unlikely out until 2007. This is only three years prior to the date set to accomplish the target, namely, to stop the increasing rates of obesity in those under the age of 11 by 2010, critics might add. Could the deployment of appropriate healthcare ICT not help speed things up? The recently released NDST white paper, "Our health, our care, our say: a new direction for community services" sets a new path for the entire U.K. health and social care system, and confirms the vision set out in the Department of Health Green Paper, Independence, Well-being and Choice, promising a radical, and sustained shift in healthcare delivery. Health services will become more personalized contextualized, and fit into people's lives[18]. Would this vision not require the incorporation of health information strategic initiatives to facilitate the achievement of the desired goals? Should individuals at risk for diabetes and heart diseases for example have to search for this recent study published in the International Journal of Obesity identified early warning sign of artery damage, for example[19]? A research team from Warwick Medical School found a link between levels of sE-selectin that indicates damage to blood vessels, and a person's weight, findings that they noted show possible use of the marker as an early indicator of artery disease. Obesity experts agreed, noting that it could indicate a new avenue of research into identifying high-risk persons and informing them. The researchers noted the importance of identifying early signs of damage, such as blocked and narrowed arteries, which can precede heart disease or stroke. They studied 260 healthy men and women of Asian, African and white ethnic origins, to examine a range of measures of obesity or fatness such as body mass index (BMI) and waist-hip ratio. The study showed a significant association between the levels of sE-selectin, a marker of inflammation produced by artery vessel walls, and measures of obesity, particularly, with the amount of fat around the waist, every 2% increase in sE-selectin linked to the increase of one unit in BMI and 0.01 units in waist-hip ratio, the findings observed in each ethnic group. According to Professor Francesco Cappuccio, one of the researchers, "This study highlights the importance of the activation of the endothelium, the inner layer of the artery vessel wall, in the metabolic processes leading to obesity and cardiovascular disease .this observation opens opportunities to develop new treatments that deal directly with inflammation either through diet or drugs". There is no doubt that understanding that this inflammation could directly set off thrombosis, heart disease, strokes, and diabetes, would make a difference to adherence to the suggestion of researches that a healthy diet could reduce levels of sE-selectin. Knowing also that some of the benefits of cholesterol-lowering statins probably result from their effects on levels of the marker would encourage medication compliance. As Professor Steve Bloom, an obesity expert at Imperial College London, noted " It would be useful to be able to identify people to tell them they are at risk, so they are able to take more exercise and watch their diet, rather than the 'blunderbuss' approach we have at the moment in terms of giving healthy living advice." Does this not articulate the need for targeted health information? IST project ePerSpace is a partnership of 19 of organizations from industry and academia. With a presentation of its integrated service management platform for the home of the future, with personalized, value-added networked services in future capable of linking all one's electronic devices in a single network, monitored and adjusted from a single point at home or anywhere, at the ongoing CeBit fair, the opportunities for targeted health information continue to rise. The researchers will also demonstrate the platform's versatility in circumstances resembling real-life situations at a workshop in Madrid on April 06, 2006. Such a platform could result in a number of new services, which earlier could not have been possible. To underscore this point, the Madrid presentation by experts from telecoms network operators France Telecom, Telefonica, and Telenor, in a workshop to the wider research community, will include live demonstrations of the technical challenges of home-network platform design, novel services that the project identified, and a business analysis of home networking applications[20]. In September 2005 in Amsterdam, ePerSpace demonstrated personalized TV services at the IBC 2005, the world s largest event for content creation and delivery, part of the NAVSHP IST village that the IST project AVISTA organized. Focused on the seamless delivery of personalized services at home, the project would likely offer immense opportunities for the delivery of targeted health information in the near future. The major thrust of the demonstration was the residential gateway on which the personal profiles reside, profiles used to deliver personalized news and TV via the gateway, making it possible to deliver personalized services, for example, health news and analyzed current health information as they emerge to the user/ subscriber, based on his/ her preferences. The demonstration of My TV, a broadcast TV program highlighted those program blocks within user profiles that support programmed recording and playback via the personal video recorder (PVR), and options to adapt content to the capabilities of the preferred receiving device, for example a PDA. The user profile is not self-learning based on monitoring usage pattern and user behavior. Rather, it needs explicit consent to update the profile, the program ensuring that the profile is strictly user controlled, content providers, and services having only access to the required information. It also offers other similar or random content items, outside the user s interest profile thus preventing an overly narrow user focus and content consumption. This project no doubt ushers in new frontiers for multimedia networking that would likely find widespread applications in the health industry including as noted earlier, in delivering targeted current and analyzed health information, with enormous potential for disease prevention, health promotion, and curative aspects of healthcare delivery among others. It also underscores the need to track emerging healthcare ICT, whose likely increasing role in different facets of healthcare delivery few would contend. Would a subscriber to such information on diabetes not benefit for example from new research findings on as benign an activity as eating potatoes, on the risk for developing Type 2 according to the results of a prospective study reported in the February 2006 issue of the *American Journal of Clinical Nutrition*? Thomas L. Halton, MD, from Harvard Medical School, Brigham, and Women's Hospital in Boston, Mass, and colleagues who carried out this study noted, "The role of potatoes in a diet aimed at reducing the burden of chronic disease has been controversial"[21]. They added, "Potatoes, a high glycemic form of carbohydrate, are hypothesized to increase insulin resistance and risk of type 2 diabetes." The study, initiated in 1976 started out with 121 700 registered female nurses, was a prospective study of 84 555 of the women, aged 34 to 59 years, with no history of chronic disease, enrolled in the Nurses' Health Study, who completed a validated food frequency questionnaire (FFQ) at baseline, and repeated dietary evaluations over a 20-year period. Four thousand, four hundred and ninety six participants received the diagnosis of type 2 diabetes, potato, and French fry consumption, positively associated with risk for type-2 diabetes, after adjustment for age and dietary and nondietary factors. The link between potato consumption and risk for type 2 diabetes in obese and sedentary women was even more significant, subgroups thought likelier to have underlying insulin resistance, which may increase the adverse metabolic effects of higher glycemic carbohydrates. The link was also more significant, "When potatoes were substituted for whole grains", the researchers also noted, and that the study limitations included the inability to detach fully, the effects of potatoes and French fries from those of the overall Western dietary pattern. Could the receipt of such information not help an at-risk person restrict his/her consumption of these foods in order to reduce the risk of type 2 diabetes or indeed, substitute these sources of carbohydrate with lower glycemic, high-fiber forms, such as whole grains, which the researchers recommended? Could this knowledge and the appropriate actions taken not help reduce the prevalence of diabetes in the U.K, and their complications, and overall health spending?

Healthcare ICT is also making significant impact on secondary prevention, specifically, the early diagnosis and prompt treatment of diseases, including ensuring patient safety in the process. Medical errors pose a major threat to patient safety, causing 44,000 98,000 deaths per year, for example in the U.S., more deaths than highway accidents, breast cancer, or AIDS cause[22]. The main cause of error-related inpatient deaths is adverse drug events (ADEs) such as medication errors, an estimated 7,000 deaths per year linked medication errors[23]. Medication errors that result in preventable ADEs could be at any stage of the medication-use process, for example according to some studies, 56%, 6%, 4%, and 34%, in the ordering, transcribing, dispensing, and administration stages, respectively[24]. An increasing number of Healthcare ICT could help reduce the rates of medication errors, for example, computerized physician order entry (CPOE), which could help prevent ordering and transcription errors. Robotics and automated drug-dispensing systems could help reduce dispensing errors. Point of care (POC) devices, for example, bar-code point-of-care (BPOC) could minimize administration errors[25]. BPOC, for example, ensures the administration of the right drug via the right route to the right patient in the right amount at the right time, termed the "five rights" of drug administration, and research evidence supports its effectiveness in preventing medication administration errors although only used in about 2% of U.S. hospitals. Could the more widespread use of this technology, including in the U.K not significantly minimize such errors, with information encoded in bar codes enabling the matching of the medication administered with the doctor's order for the patient? Underlying the ultimate goal of any health system, including the U.K health system should be the provision of comprehensive and qualitative health services to all whether or not they have to pay fully or partially for it. The argument regarding financing health services seems moot in a dispensation where their increasing costs are becoming too burdensome for all stakeholders, while simultaneously, the public expects increasingly more from the health services. There is no doubt that a number of factors determine health-financing model, but equally none that resources are exhaustible, which means that both publicly and privately funded health systems, or countries that have a mix of both must seek ways to rationalize healthcare spending, which the appropriate deployment of healthcare ICT could help achieve. Canada, for example officially is the only industrialized country that bars private clinics legally from providing services covered by the public system, even though many in practice do so. However, the country's health system is at the brink of fundamental changes, some would contend, with the recent Supreme Court decision in Quebec essentially ruling that the province should allow private healthcare services to operate, and with Alberta recently announcing plans to proceed with its "Third Way" model, which would enable delivery of more health services by the private sector. Quebec announced its own plans earlier, British Columbia s on the way. There are of course concerns among those against these developments, while those that support them believe that there is no other way forward for an increasingly too-costly-to-maintain public health system. The question, however, really is whether healthcare delivery would meet the ideals of the Canada Health Act, including the provision of accessible, comprehensive, portable, qualitative, and well-governed health system. Regardless of whether such a health system is publicly-or privately funded, healthcare ICT is critical for achieving these laudable goals. Important to recognize also is the fact that it is easier and less costly to prevent many of the diseases that create the economic burden on health systems in many countries today, including the U.K, and again, healthcare ICT could play a major role in achieving this goal. Indeed, some experts believe that the curative healthcare delivery model is simply unsustainable in contemporary times. The vision of the director of the U.S National Institute of Health (NIH), Elias Zerhouni, M.D., for example is for a fundamental paradigm shift in the practice of medicine and that only scientific innovation could make this happen, which he articulated in an interview published today on the *Health Affairs* Web site on March 9, 2006[26]. Zerhouni notes that electronic medical records (EMR) and national health insurance could help reduce medical costs, albeit it marginally, but that the country really needs scientific innovation that facilitates earlier intervention in the disease process describing his job as being " a provocateur, not a manager of the status quo." Much like the prevailing health zeitgeist, the director again emphasizes the crucial need for adopting a preventive health model and the role that technological innovation could play in its materialization. Indeed, Zerhouni also stresses intersectoral collaboration and knowledge convergence and lists nanotechnology, clinical databases designed to answer research questions, systems biology, and openness to radical ideas, being among his top priorities, and plans to leverage NIH funding in order to spend money more wisely and such that it has a cumulative positive effect on population health. Does any contemporary health system including in the U.K, not need to adopt a preventive population health approach, backed by technological innovation to remain viable, and could a health system survive otherwise? Is it inevitable that health systems worldwide move in the direction of healthcare costs prudence, in the face of soaring health spending, which some argue, does not deliver on its promise of qualitative health, anyway? Why does health spending continue to increase in many countries, including in the U.K, a clearly unsustainable state of affairs if the health system did not need reviewing, perhaps with unconventional lenses? Could it be that these countries are not exploiting to the hilt, the opportunities healthcare ICT offer, to help reduce transaction costs, for example? Should we not be even considering ensuring that diseases do not even occur in the first place, not even those we do not know currently exist? Information technologies are opening our eyes to the biology of the gene, with active research on genomics and proteomics capable of equipping us with knowledge that could make it possible to figure the variety of ways that an individual's bodily organs could go wrong, and at what points in the person's life. Innovative technologies could even offer preemptive options for stopping the flaws from occurring let alone manifesting in the individual. Would investing in such innovative technologies now not pay off in future? What opportunities for excellence, could nurturing a healthy future generation create for further innovations and the future of humankind? It is impossible to discard curative medicine altogether, now, or even in future, except of course we are able to arrive at a perfect knowledge of the various interplay of the innumerable systems operational in nature. This seems on the surface Herculean, but we could achieve it by first creating the sort of necessary increasingly enabling milieu that taking health matters seriously would create, including investing in innovative health information and other technologies that could further improve our knowledge and practice of healthcare delivery. While we contemplate the future, we need to remember the here and now, and seek ways to address effectively the immediate problems confronting the health system, which include the excessive costs of curative medicine. This is where the benefits derivable from the widespread deployment of health information technologies, for example, electronic health records (EHR) in tackling these problems even if marginal in the short, and medium terms, would add up to substantial proportions in the long term, and significantly help reduce healthcare spending while simultaneously improving the quality of healthcare delivery. One of the key roles of healthcare ICT in healthcare delivery is enabling the communication and sharing of health information. There is no doubt about the importance of an efficient conduct of these activities in facilitating qualitative, perhaps even life saving healthcare delivery at the point of care (POC). As the example given earlier of a U.K resident vacationing in Europe, the availability of accurate, and timely information on the individual's health, for example, that he/ she has high blood pressure, and the medication, allergy, and drug interaction histories, could make the difference between life and death in an ER in say Vienna, the person comatose. In other words, the U.K health system not only needs to have a nationwide health information network and promote its widespread adoption and interoperability among providers in and outside the NHS, but also must work towards cross-border interconnectivity of such health information networks. Healthcare spending in the U.K as a percentage of its gross domestic product (GDP) in 1997 was 6.8% and continues to increase, more than £ 67 billion in 2002, 7.7% of the GDP and 8% up on 2001, the pattern continuing. The government's inclusive spending review, published in September 2002, allocated a steady rise in spending to the NHS, expected to increase from £ 65.4bn ($109bn; €95bn) in 2002-03 to £ 105.6bn in 2007-8, an average year on year real growth of about 7.4%. Furthermore, health spending in the U.K is increasing faster in England than other parts of the country, over the past six years, with even the gap between England Scotland, Wales, and Northern Ireland, all that customarily spent more per person than England, narrowed. A Northern office of the Institute of Public Policy Research and the Economic and Social Research Council reports indicates that health spending in England rose by 65% between 1999-2001 and 2004-5, compared with increases of 47% in Wales, 43% in Northern Ireland, and 38% in Scotland during the same period. Meanwhile, devolution has resulted in more divergence in health policy across the country, with the four countries pursuing disparate healthcare priorities, just when the public expects common standards of public services across the U.K. An example of such expectations is the concept of patient-led NHS, with emphasis on not just meeting the practical and physical aspects of patient care but also patients' emotional needs. The NHS plans to improve upon simply achieving the Public Service Agreement (PSA), and to pay attention to the expectations of patients at an emotional level, in other words, to how patients feel about their experience of using the NHS and what they value, treating patients with dignity and respect. Providing patients with required information, for example, on how much longer, they would be on a surgical wait list, rather than not, leaving them feeling ignored, even abandoned, would likely improve the individual's emotional experience of service provision despite the wait. The crucial factor is for such goals to be consistent right through the country, which again would require information technology-backed coordination of standards across the country. Indeed, the NHS Improvement Plan, published in June 2004, which established how the NHS needs to change to become truly patient-led notes that the next stage in the NHS's journey is: "to ensure that a drive for responsive, convenient and personalized services takes root across the whole NHS and for all patients. For hospital services, this means that there will be a lot more choice for patients about how, when, and where they are treated and much better information to support that." The document also notes that "From the end of 2005, patients will have the right to choose from at least four to five different healthcare providers, and the right to choose from any provider as long as they meet clear NHS standards." "Creating a Patient-led NHS", published in March 2005, built on the theme of delivering a patient-led NHS, underscoring the increasing importance of "patient choice" in health service provision, but as earlier noted, how could patients make rational choices when they lack current, accurate, and timely information to help in so doing? The NHS plans to give healthcare providers incentives to offer care that is efficient, responsive, of a high standard and respects people's dignity, attributes of care that would improve the patient's emotional experience. However, is the NHS planning to offer them incentives to implement healthcare ICT, which is critical for providing patients with the information that would help improve their emotional experience of service delivery, which itself hinges on making the right choices regarding service provision? Regardless of whether the healthcare delivery model is consumer-driven, as is the direction it seems headed in the U.S or patient-led as it is, in the U.K, health systems with different funding philosophies, it is obvious that the patient or consumer is now at the center of the healthcare delivery world. Patient-focused concepts such as the freedom to choose providers, emotional experience, respect and dignity, have become important elements in healthcare delivery, bringing the need for healthcare ICT-backed, communication of targeted health information, health information sharing, and availability in real time at the point of care squarely to the fore. Would it not be essential therefore for health policy planning in the U.K to incorporate this convergence of information technologies and health information and knowledge base into the vision of healthcare delivery in the country, besides addressing the short-and medium terms health problems with the implementation of appropriate healthcare ICT as necessary? It is certainly possible for the NHS to achieve its core values of providing equal access to care that is available at the point of need regardless of ability to pay, personal to the individual patient and achieved within a taxpayer-funded system that must demonstrate value for money. The question of whether it must remain tax-funded, or embrace private health insurance and to what extent remains moot. Not least because either way, health information technologies are going to play a major role in integrating the supply-side, demand-side, transactional and systems management reform goals the NHS has set for itself in order to meet the ever-increasing public demand for it to deliver on its promise to achieve its core values. Giving patients and users more choice, providers more freedom to innovate and, to compete against one another and embracing fiscal discipline in the health system all require significant investments in information technologies to achieve. It is probably safe to say that the overall benefits of these technologies to the wellbeing of the public and the economy of the country will most certainly offset, sooner than later, their costs.

References

1. Halbower AC, Marcus CL. Sleep Disorders in Children. *Curr Opin Pulm Med* 9(6):471-476, 2003. © 2003 Lippincott Williams & Wilkins

2. Mahowald MW, Kader G, Schenck CH. Clinical categories of sleep disorders I. Continuum 1997;3:35-65.

3. Karni A, Tanne D, Rubenstein BS, Askenasy JJ, Sagi D. Dependence on REM sleep of overnight improvement of a perceptual skill. *Science*. 1994; 265:679-682

4. Available at: http://www.sensation-eu.org/
Accessed on March 07, 2006

5. Available at:
http://www.temple.edu/news_media/documents/study_article_Bass_3.pdf
Accessed on March 08, 2006

6. Available at: http://www.cato.org/pub_display.php?pub_id=5871
Accessed on March 08, 2006

7. Available at: http://www.medscape.com/viewarticle/523538?src=mp Accessed on March 09, 2006

8. Available at: http://www.medscape.com/viewarticle/524455?src=mp Accessed on March 09, 2006

9. Agency for Healthcare Research and Quality. Comparative effectiveness of management strategies for gastroesophageal reflux disease. Rockville, Md: Agency for Healthcare Research and Quality; December 2005. Available at:

http://effectivehealthcare.ahrq.gov/synthesize/reports/final.cfm?Document=2&Topic=30 Accessed March 9, 2006

10. Available at: http://www.nytimes.com/2006/03/10/national/10aging.html?_r=2&oref=slogin&oref=slogin Accessed on March 10, 2006

11. Bingham SA et al. *Lancet* 2003; 361: 1496-501

12. Parks et al. JAMA 2005; 294: 2849-57

13. Available at: http://www.diabetes.nhs.uk/ Accessed on March 10, 2006

14. Available at: http://www.timesonline.co.uk/article/0,,2091-2059194,00.html Accessed on March 10, 2006

15. Available at: http://www.telegraph.co.uk/news/main.jhtml?xml=/news/2006/02/26/ndiab26.xml&sSheet=/news/2006/02/26/ixnewstop.html. Accessed on March 10, 2006

16. Available at: www.diabetes.org.uk/news/feb06/MORI_results.doc Accessed on March 10, 2006

17. Available at: http://news.bbc.co.uk/2/hi/health/4756370.stm Accessed on March 10, 2006

18. Available at: http://www.diabetes.nhs.uk/downloads/our_health_our_care_full_version.pdf Accessed on March 10, 2006

19. Available at: http://news.bbc.co.uk/go/pr/fr/-/2/hi/health/4780326.stm Accessed on March 10, 2006

20. Available at: http://www.ist-eperspace.org/ Accessed on March 11, 2006

21. *Am J Clin Nutr.* 2006; 83:284-290

22. Kohn LT, Corrigan JM, Donaldson MS, eds. To err is human: building a safer health system. Washington, DC: National Academy Press; 1999.

23. Migdial K. Medication errors: the scope of the problem. www.ahrq.gov/qual/ Accessed on March 11, 2006

24. Bates DW, Cullen DJ, Laird N et al. Incidence of adverse drug events and potential adverse drug events. Implications for prevention. *JAMA*. 1995; 274:29-34.

25. Winterstein AG, Johns TE, Rosenberg EI et al. Nature and causes of clinically significant medication errors in a tertiary care hospital. *Am J Health-Syst Pharm*. 2004; 61:1908-16.

26. Available at: http://content.healthaffairs.org/cgi/reprint/hlthaff.25.w94v1 Accessed on March 11, 2006

27. Available at: http://bmj.bmjjournals.com/ Accessed on March 11, 2006

Canada Health System Revisited

Healthcare delivery in Canada seems to be at a turning point. There is the crucial issue of whether the country should have a parallel private health system, the call by some given legal teeth by the Supreme Court ruling in 2005 that Quebec residents could seek private healthcare. The province announced some measures guaranteeing limited private healthcare delivery in early 2006. Alberta also announced its "Third Way" healthcare delivery model, a step closer to full private healthcare delivery in the province, and British Columbia's plans are in the offing. Private firms are setting up private healthcare services in different parts of the country. The momentum seems to be increasing rapidly as the debate heats up. A key issue in the debate on the future of healthcare delivery in Canada is clearly funding-related, and justifiably so. With the country's healthcare spending ever increasing, it is becoming increasingly clear that this copious spending on health is not just alarming, but also unsustainable. Even those that contend that the provinces and territories, which statutorily manage health services, might just still appear to be coping because they are receiving increasing federal largesse, concede that not only is that support less sufficient to meet the demands on health services, but that they are fully aware that the country may not have a budget surplus indefinitely. In other words, the stage is set for an imperative wager on the direction the country's health system will head. Health expenditure as a percentage of Gross domestic products (GDP) in Canada in 1990 was 9.05%, total health expenditures per capita in U.S dollars during the same year, 1945. Canada's Capital spending on health has also been increasing over the years, more than doubling in the past seven years (1996-2003), indicative of significant investments in high-tech equipment such as MRIs and CT scanners, and on new buildings. The country planned to infuse approximately $41 billion into its health system over a decade, and in its 2005 health budget, to add $2.5 billion to the Canada Health Transfer, increasing the base to $19 billion, itself expected to increase yearly by six percent, as embodied in the "escalator clause". Based on 2004 estimates, and at $31,500, Canada had the 12th highest GDP in the world, compared to the global average of $8,800, and those for the US and the UK, $40,100, 2nd highest, and $29,600, 16th highest, respectively, expressed on a purchasing power parity (PPP) basis and divided by population as of 1 July for the same year. These estimates are in US funds. According to the Canadian Institute for Health Information (CIHI), Canada's total health expenditures were $121.4 billion in 2003, a real (inflation-adjusted) increase of 4.6% over 2002, akin to the increase (4.5%) estimated for 2002. This rate of growth was down from the increases of more than 5% per year seen from 1996 to 2001 but was enough to increase health spending to an estimated 10% of Canada's Gross Domestic Product (GDP). In 2001, Canada's health spending as a proportion of its GDP was 9.7%, behind the US at 13.9%, Switzerland at 11.1%, and Germany at 10.7%, and in 2002 and 2003, it ranked fourth among a list of 12 comparative Organization for Economic Cooperation and Development (OECD) countries on the same parameter. Estimates of Canada's health care spending for 2005 were $142.0 billion, a 7.7% increase over 2004, and a real increase of 5.0%, after adjusting for inflation, according to the CIHI annual report on health care spending in Canada, National Health Expenditure Trends 1975 2005 released on December 17, 2005[1]. The new estimates also noted the continuing rise in health care spending as a percentage of GDP, for example from 7% in 1975, to 10.0% by 1992, rising again to an estimated 10.4% in 2004, an all-time high, after a gradual fall to 8.9% in 1996. Indeed, the country's health spending has in the last several years, been growing faster than its economy, which some attribute, partly, to funds devoted in the last several health accords the provinces and territories are now receiving. Nonetheless, the increasing healthcare spending is having many wonder if not, at some point, if not now, the country would have to take certain fundamental decisions on this issue. Considering the passion that envelopes different viewpoints on this and other core issues confronting the country's health system, just when and if any dramatic change to the health system will occur is, for now, conjectural. Recent developments in Ontario exemplify the dimensions of the issues involved in re-charting the path of healthcare delivery in the country. Queen's Park has approved the far-reaching legislation to reform Ontario's healthcare system, yet the controversy over the Local Health Integration Act, a first step in major changes to healthcare delivery in the province, persists, in particular, firmly opposed by labor unions and nurses. The bill, likely soon passed, creates 14 regional authorities, termed local health integration networks, across the province, and not unlike the health boards of other provinces each network responsible for co-

coordinating health-care services within its jurisdiction, the networks, controlling $20 billion in health spending, over half of Ontario s total health-care budget. The idea of the budget is to decentralize decision-making on health services and promote their control at the local level, based on the assumption that it is best to determine community's health-care service needs at the local level where their delivery occurs. In other words, rather than having such decisions made at Queen's Park, the health-care officials and practitioners at the local networks will do so, and are best positioned to ensure patients receive a continuum of healthcare from diagnosis, through treatment, recovery and rehabilitation. Labor unions and other critics hold that the plan will result in hospital closures, hence job losses, because service rationalization to exploit economies of scale would result in certain services no longer offered at some hospitals, but centralized at other health facilities in the network, while retaining minimal essential service levels. Proponents contend that the province needs to act with its health-care costs increasing yearly, more than the inflation rate, guzzling 50% of its budget and that the government deserves credit for taking measures to reduce this escalating rate and to spend public funds more judiciously[2]. The bill also provides for competitive bidding in local health services provision, which some argue would enable private health-care providers, perhaps offering lower wages and benefits, to underbid non-profit agencies that provided community services in the past, citing the increasing prominence of for-profit providers in operating the new provincially-funded long-term care beds in the past six years. There are those opposed to other aspects of the bill, including those pertaining to changing the geographical boundaries of the networks, despite government reassurance to protect the non-profit sector's continuing participation in healthcare delivery in the province. The reform plans of Alberta and British Columbia also face challenges. Premier Gordon Campbell of British Columbia recently committed B.C. to a three-year discussion of health change and "updating" the Canada Health Act in order to "strengthen" it. Just as Alberta did a few years ago, British Columbia intends to codify the five principles of the Canada Health Act provincially a move critics deem an indirect approach to privatizing the province's health services, toward an American-style system[3]. Should it indeed matter to patients whether they receive treatment in public or private facilities, if publicly paid for, some would ask? Does private healthcare delivery signal the end of Medicare? Some people might not care about removing a troublesome appendix electively, preferring to wait until acutely indicated, while others want to be back in form promptly, and would rather not join a hospital wait list. In any case, do workers' compensation packages not take care of why the latter kind might prefer private health care? This is the same reason, its flipside, that some believe that the public health system is in jeopardy, people requesting magnetic resonance imaging each time they sprain their ankle, increasing costs, there being no adverse selection, or cost sharing. Are these increasing costs sustainable? Should government not ponder over the health spending increase that its aging population would incur? Does this not call for fiscal prudence? How could healthcare ICT help in achieving such prudence, and does it really matter whether the health system is private or public for healthcare ICT to do so? Recent healthcare ICT-backed innovations, in Alberta and Saskatchewan, for examples, indicate that the public system could reduce wait lists to weeks. Would this encourage the demand for private healthcare? Some in fact, do not see a future for private health system in Canada, arguing that its expensive premiums would discourage people, except perhaps some young or healthy people who would pay the costly premiums, which as with life or disability insurance, denied those diagnosed with some disease. Recent polls suggest Albertans want to maintain the status quo. Some are sure about the replication in the near future of the Supreme Court decision in other provinces. Others are already asking, if equality means that everyone endures the same long wait to receive healthcare, or if barring access to private care is a reasonable limit on life and liberty, considering American-style, constitutional protection. Yet, is it not possible that exploring the immense opportunities progress in healthcare information technologies offer for their applications in various aspects of healthcare delivery, would make the funding model of healthcare provision irrelevant? Would it make competition universal, that is not just among private healthcare providers but also between the private and public health sectors that consumers are able to choose their healthcare providers? Would such competition bring down healthcare costs? Could it be such that government would not pay for both private and public healthcare provision, minimizing the chances of those that could afford private health insurance swelling healthcare costs utilizing public services at their convenience, leaving the rest of the people jostling for places on a longer wait lists, increasing morbidities, and worsening health spending? What could more rational medication-prescribing do to reduce healthcare costs, and how could healthcare ICT, for example, computerized physician order entry (CPOE) and bar-coding technologies help in this regard? Would it not be necessary for patients to have current, accurate, and timely health information in order to make sound judgment regarding choice of providers? Would being able to make such sound judgment make healthcare consumers more discerning, in particular if they paid part of the costs of health services provision? What would government speeding up approval for less expensive yet effective medications do to help reduce healthcare costs? Should patients not participate in decisions regarding the medications they receive, for example, between brands and generics? How would having knowledge of the differences between them help in making such decisions, and how could healthcare ICT help furnish them with such knowledge? There is no doubt that the answers to these and other relevant questions would help clarify even more the issues involved in the future direction of healthcare delivery in Canada. That the country is investing substantially in healthcare ICT speaks to its belief in the value of these technologies in improving healthcare delivery, and in reducing healthcare spending. Yet, it does not seem that all healthcare stakeholders either agree or appreciate that the benefits derivable from the applications of these technologies in the health industry are legion, and by far would offset the investments incurred implementing them, in the long-if not the short-term, or how else could one explain the slowness of healthcare providers in embracing these technologies? Could healthcare not duplicate the gains that information technologies enabled in other industries? Indeed, what is the worth of healthcare ICT diffusion to health in particular and to society, and what should government do, if anything, to accelerate its widespread adoption in the health system?

Recently, Health Canada issued an advisory on the link that a recent study found between the selective serotonin reuptake inhibitors (SSRIs) and a condition called persistent pulmonary hypertension of the newborn (PPHN), sometimes called persistent fetal circulation (PFC) in babies born to women who took these medications, used mostly to treat depression, during the second half of their pregnancies[4]. Health Canada is requesting women to discuss the issue with their doctors, but emphasizing that they should not stop taking their medication without first consulting their doctor. PPHN, which essentially shunts blood away from the baby's lungs, into the fetal circulation, is comparatively rare but clearly life threatening, and associated with substantial morbidity and mortality. The study, published in the February 9, 2006 issue of the New England Journal of Medicine, noted that babies born with this condition were six times more likely than healthy babies to have had exposures to SSRIs, such as those Health Canada mentioned, namely, Wellbutrin (bupropion); Celexa (citalopram); Cipralex (escitalopram); Prozac (fluoxetine); Luvox (fluvoxamine); Remeron (mirtazapine); Paxil (paroxetine); Zoloft (sertraline). Others include, Effexor (venlafaxine) and Zyban (bupropion), also prescribed for smoking cessation. The researchers noted that a previous cohort study suggested a possible link between maternal use of the SSRI fluoxetine late in the third trimester of pregnancy and the risk of PPHN in the infant. They conducted a case-control study between 1998 and 2003, to determine whether there is a link between PPHN and exposure to SSRIs during late pregnancy, with 377 women whose infants had PPHN and 836 matched control women and their infants, enrolled. Nurse, blind to the study hypothesis re medication use in pregnancy and likely confounders, including demographic variables and health history, conducted the maternal interviews. The researchers found exposure to an SSRI in 14 infants with PPHN after the completion of the 20th week of gestation, compared with six control infants. On the other hand, they found no association between SSRI use, prior to the 20th week of gestation, or the use of non-SSRI antidepressant drugs at any time during pregnancy, and higher PPHN risk, hence concluded, that there is an association between the maternal use of SSRIs in late pregnancy and PPHN in the offspring. Although they suggested further investigation, the authors noted the need for caution in the use of SSRIs in pregnancy, which is essentially, what Health Canada, also wanted women to know, although it is another matter how. This example underscores the need for targeted healthcare ICT-enabled health information as part of such efforts to get crucial health information to reach those that need them in a timely and effective fashion. There is no doubt that some women would have heard about the Health Canada advisory in the news, or read about it on the Internet, or perhaps heard about it via their doctors, but there is likely to be many others who have not, some of whom might currently be pregnant and on one or the other SSRI. To highlight the concern of Health

Canada regarding this issue, it stated in the advisory that SSRI treatment should only persist if the benefits to the patient outweighed the risks to the fetus, also noting the association with SSRI use of an increase in the overall risk of major birth defects. What could be the emotional costs to a new mother of her bay developing these complications, if it survived and to the baby over a lifetime, not to mention costs to the health system of increased resource utilization by both, the advisory not reaching such a woman when pregnant? Should we therefore not be concerned about ensuring that women indeed receive this advisory, rather expecting them to seek the information, or hope that they would be watching the evening news on TV? Could we not prevent many other diseases by ensuring that crucial health information reaches its target? Could such prevention efforts, which healthcare ICT could not only facilitate but also cost-effectively, not help reduce overall health spending in the end? Would it matter if women received the advisory via the public or private health system? On the other hand, all stakeholders have the responsibility to ensure that such crucial health information reaches the targeted audience. Would it not be faster, cheaper, and more efficient to send such information via an e-mail, instant messenger, or other electronic format, its contents and format tailored to the targeted audience, than via snail mail? Would individuals encouraged to have personal health records (PHR), into which they could authorize the delivery of targeted health information, not facilitate health education campaigns of this sort? Could the widespread diffusion of electronic health records, not help determine who needs what information, and such information delivered to the appropriate person in real time? The point here is that the starting point of healthcare delivery is the individual, who should also be at the core of any healthcare policy, and information collection, aggregation, storage, communication and sharing are essential activities in delivering comprehensive, qualitative, accessible, and effective healthcare services to an individual. Healthcare ICT is crucial for the efficient and effective conduct of these activities, hence of their chances of enabling the achievement of the critical goal of healthcare delivery to the individual. The achievement of this goal serves not just the purpose of nurturing a healthier, and more productive populace, but also that of curtailing health spending without compromising the quality of healthcare delivery, yet freeing scarce resources for deployment in other key areas. In other words, we need to come to terms with the fact that health is one of the most information intensive industries, information that not just accumulates in the course of an individual's overall health history, but because of the progress in medical knowledge and in related fields, including information and communications technologies. Furthermore, we should actually encourage information creation and flow in the industry, as this improves our understanding and sharpens our management of diseases and other aspects of healthcare delivery. Consider this. A recent study published in the March 13, 2006, issue of "Cancer Cell" sshows that researchers have found a unique molecular profile for lung cancer. The researchers found that the expression pattern of certain microRNAs, or miRNAs, might predict tumor aggressiveness in some patients with lung cancer, findings that indicate that miRNAs may represent a new class of diagnostic and prognostic tools for lung cancer. miRNAs are tiny segments of genetic material called ribonucleic acid, or RNA that control gene expression, hence whose actions could change the expression of cancer-related genes within a cell and result in malignancies. The researchers identified two miRNAs, namely, "has-mir-155" and "has-let-7a-2" valuable as prognostic indicators in patients with adenocarcinoma, a malignancy of pulmonary mucous glands, high and low levels of the former and latter respectively linked with poor disease outcome, the former, signaling of the miRNA to change the amount of a protein produced, more significant, regardless of tumor stage. The levels of these biomarkers for an individual would indicate more or less intense treatment of a tumor, help with treatment planning, and offer realistic expectations of possible outcomes, independent of tumor stage. According to Curtis Harris, M.D., chief of the Laboratory of Human Carcinogenesis at NCI and co-leader of this study, "Following surgery, 50 to 60 percent of patients with stage I lung cancer will develop metastatic disease within five years, (which) may indicate that there are micrometastases that have not been detected by imaging, scanning or pathology." He added, "in the future, we can use miRNAs and other biological predictors to select patients who may need more aggressive treatment versus those who may not. Additional studies confirming these results are the next step before incorporating miRNA analysis into routine clinical practice." Lung cancer is one of the main causes of death due to cancer, exposure to tobacco smoke, its primary cause. However, some people that have never smoked cigarettes also develop the disease, which makes the findings of this study the more significant as they could help unravel the mechanisms underlying this disease, besides miRNAs also providing opportunities to examine the regulation of cancer-related genes. "miRNAs are going to be important biomarkers of not only diagnosis and prognosis, but therapy, as well," said Harris, adding ",The next step is to identify the genes that the miRNAs are affecting; they could be used as potential targets for developing novel therapies." Several other studies indicate that other types of cancers express specific miRNAs, but the precise role that miRNAs play in the development of human cancers is unknown, although a recent paper in the Proceedings of the National Academy of Science gave credence to the observation of the regulation of cancer-related genes by miRNAs in solid tumors[6]. Should governments participate directly or via collaborative efforts with research and private sector organizations to invest in such knowledge generation as part of its strategic vision of the future of the country s healthcare delivery? Would investing in such research endeavors not perhaps ultimately enable us understand the constitution of the human organisms enough to personalize healthcare delivery, including pre-empting illness, rather than simply preventing disease? In other words, to know that certain cellular reactions might result in some "flaws", and stop that happening, that is from progressing to a "disease", hitherto unknown? Should strategic investments in medical research and technology, including healthcare ICT, therefore not be an important dimension of contemporary approaches to conceptualizing healthcare delivery in Canada? How could the country s health budget benefit from the findings of the research mentioned above, for example, with the reduction in morbidities and mortalities they could engender? Could one safely conclude that the benefits of such strategic investments sometimes are in the medium, if not short-, rather than long-terms, making the returns on investments even more palpable? Would the quality of care delivered by healthcare providers not improve significantly armed with current and timely information such as those of the research findings? Would it not be necessary to develop appropriate healthcare ICT-backed approaches for delivering such information targeted at the practitioners that need them, contextualized, perhaps even analyzed in the appropriate format that the practitioner opted for signing up for such a service? Could private organizations not in fact establish such services to which healthcare providers could subscribe, making it unnecessary for providers to have to scavenge for required information, on top of their busy schedules, in complicated databases that come up with an information glut for a simple keyword search? Considering that information acquisition is the first in a series of activities crucial to the normal and effective operations of an information-intensive industry, such as the health industry, there cannot be any gainsaying the need for information technologies that would enable targeted health information dissemination.

Indeed, not just healthcare professionals need health information, all healthcare stakeholders do. Patients and other individuals are becoming increasingly interested in acquiring health information, which helps them in a number of ways, including to understand the diseases from which they or people they know suffer, and in enabling them to make the right choices about their healthcare providers, and to participate meaningfully in decisions regarding their health, in short, empowering them. This seems to be the inevitable direction of healthcare delivery, and is one that has spawned novel healthcare-delivery models, such as consumer-driven healthcare in the U.S, and patient-led health in the U.K. It seems reasonable to expect that the public would be placing increasing demands on health services the more information it has on health issues, in particular, on current and new discoveries such as the findings relating to lung cancer mentioned above, or that to PPHN or any new research findings delivered to individuals via targeted health information technologies. However, this is true on to a certain degree, in fact, only in the short term, which is a good thing for both the individual and for government. In the short term, individuals would be more acutely aware of the treatment options that they have, and demand it from their healthcare providers. Let us assume that Medicare remains the main source of healthcare provision for its peoples, this could result in even more health spending, as patients seek investigations and treatments that are more sophisticated since adverse selection does not operate, and everyone has access to healthcare, except of course government devices an effective means to minimize resource over-utilization. Meantime, the acquisition of healthcare ICT-backed health information, personalized and via public health campaigns, would buoy health promotion and disease prevention, particularly, and even if only over time, as the young people who literally would have grown up with such information if targeted at early in life, become older, and healthier than the preceding generations. This means lesser and lesser pressure on the health system with time for treatment purposes. Imagine what would happen were we in fact able to pre-empt disease formation someday? The above illustrates the inherent flaw in the common argument that investing in technologies increase healthcare costs. It may seem so in the immediate term, but scrutiny would reveal that the technologies pay for themselves, literally, in the long term. In a private healthcare system, information acquisition would also increase the demand on healthcare providers to deliver the best services. This would spur competition in a free-market setting, healthcare providers implementing even more healthcare ICT to enhance their value propositions, and swell their customer base. As some argue, these information technologies would become, essentially commoditized among some providers, specifically those unwilling or incapable of creating innovative value-added services that would in tandem with the deployment of appropriate information technologies give them a competitive edge. Among these providers, the battleground would shift to prices, which in order not to out-price their practices, would fall, to equilibrium levels, given perfect, or near-perfect, market operations. Even mergers, and acquisitions, would be inadequate to prevent this progression, except of course the new, larger entities offer new and innovative value to their service profiles. Over time, the consumer would become the dominant driver of qualitative changes in health service provision. There is another dimension to this consumer power though, that is the need for them to be increasingly discerning in their choices of healthcare providers and services if they paid part of their healthcare costs. This added dimension would also depend on individuals having the necessary information and knowledge to make those choices, again highlighting the need for targeted health information delivery. Armed with such information, individuals would seek the best health services at the most affordable costs, contributing in no small measure to the eventual downward price spiral mentioned earlier. What would all these mean for such a privately funded health system? It would mean more individuals being able to afford health insurance in the long term, a healthier, population, and a reduction in health insurance and overall government health spending. Here again, there are a number of confounding factors that require, despite the need for deregulation in general, government intervention on a limited scale, for example, preventing health plan conglomeration and monopolies, which though might eventually bottom out as discussed earlier could create sufficient immediate schisms to compromise access to health services, particularly by the poor, and uninsured. In other words, healthcare ICT diffusion would also play a key role in how the dynamics among the various healthcare drivers in an essentially privately funded health system also pan out, as it would, indeed in a dual health system, such as some propose for Canada. In such a dual or two-tier health system, competitive forces would be cross-platform, operating among private healthcare providers on the one hand, and between them and the public health system on the other, in both instances, healthcare ICT defining capabilities for distinguishing service provision that would determine pricing and patronage, and ultimately, the survival or otherwise of either. In the short term, the intensity of competition would result in the establishment of sophisticated private healthcare services, which would become increasingly affordable, the public health system, gradually easing out of the race, coalescing service offerings as more people utilize the more affordable and qualitative health services. With resources freed in one area, that of hospitalization and prescription medication costs, and redeployed in basic and applied science and technology research, more intensive health education and promotion campaigns, and other population health measures, government would be making increasingly significant contributions to disease prevention and health promotion. Coupled with the improved curative services the private sector provides, the result would be an increasingly healthier and more productive populace, with gradually less health spending by government. In other words, the private sector, by necessarily ensuring its survival, would be facilitating the achievement of government s commitments to health services provision in accordance with the provisions of the Canada Health Act, albeit in tandem with the suave husbandry by both sectors of the immense opportunities that health information technologies offer. Is it therefore not prudent in many ways to recognize the central role that healthcare ICT would play in the future of healthcare delivery in Canada, and incorporate this recognition in the strategic vision of the future of the country's healthcare delivery, manifested in specific initiatives predicated on continuing analyses of the array of factors, internal, cross-border, and global, involved? Healthcare ICT is not only important in the effective and efficient capture, collation, and dissemination of targeted health information, which as the preceding discussion indicates, is a veritable health promotion, and disease prevention resource, it also plays a critical role in another aspect of health information utilization, in treating diseases.

Electronic health records systems (EHR) for example in association with a provincial, and eventually, national, health information network, make essential patient information available to healthcare providers in real time at the point of care (POC). This not only facilitates qualitative health service provision, it could be life-saving for the patient, for example, who is comatose, or otherwise unable to provide health information to an ER doctor to which he/ she presents while on a trip to say another town or province. How much could the widespread adoption of such healthcare ICT save in human and material terms in such and other circumstances? Would it be necessary for the country to examine cross-border availability of patient health information considering the heavy human traffic between it and its southern neighbor, for example? Would it not be necessary to initiate collaborative efforts to determine the logistics of such health information sharing in terms of technical issues, for example, systems interoperability, professional issues, for example, certification issues, and legal issues, among others? Should such patient information sharing not also be transatlantic, and should Canada s strategic vision for health not incorporate the inevitable interconnectivity of peoples and nations, and its possible consequences for global disease transmission? Would such global reach of patient information not facilitate the treatment of Canadians worldwide, reducing the burden of disease that the country eventually bears, and that of the citizens of other countries, enhancing the country s health services image and promoting tourism, hence the country s wealth? Would such global collaboration not help improve the health of many around the globe and reduce the chances of the development of diseases, for example, even a pandemic, that could have far-reaching consequences for countries beyond its origins? Does this not underline the multifaceted dimensions of healthcare conceptualizing that belie the major and continuing paradigm shifts in contemporary healthcare delivery, rooted in healthcare ICT, and to which Canada, as indeed, every country needs to subscribe?

An international study of 349 patients over two years presented at the 2006 American College of Cardiology meeting, held in Atlanta(March 11-14, 2006) revealed important findings that the public should know about and even delivered to targeted individuals at risk for cardiovascular diseases. The study, slated for publication in the April 2006 edition of the Journal of the American Medical Association, found that high doses of a powerful new statin, rosuvastatin might not just stall the build-up of fatty deposits inside the arterial walls, termed atherosclerosis (plaque), which could cause a number of cardiovascular diseases including heart attacks, but also actually reverse it. Two hundred and thirty three thousand people die from cardiovascular disease annually in the UK, and an estimated 16.7 million a year worldwide. Eight in ten (80%) Canadians have at least 1 risk factor for cardiovascular disease and 11%, three risk factors or more according to The Growing Burden of Heart Disease and Stroke in Canada, the sixth in a series of reports from the Canadian Heart and Stroke Surveillance System (CHSSS) published in 2003[7]. The report predicted an increase in the numbers of cases of cardiovascular diseases over the next two decades, hence also an increase in the resultant burden, in the main because of the continuing increase in some risk factors, for example, overweight, even among young people, diabetes and high blood pressure, and physical inactivity. Furthermore, the "greying of Canada" is an added factor in the increasing burden, the population aged 80 years and above, which rose between 1991 and 2001 by 41% to 932,000, expected to increase an additional 43% between 2001 and 2011, past an estimated 1.3 million. Between 1991 and 2001, the population between 45 and 64 years of age increased 36%, as the baby boomers entered into this group. The 2001 Census indicated that seniors aged 65 and over made up 13% of the Canadian population in 2001, up from almost 12% in 1991, estimated to rise to 15% by 2011 and just above 20% by 2025. Do these figures not call for an urgent policy review of the approaches to managing the increasing burden of cardiovascular diseases? Indeed, should we not be examining ways to prevent them in the first place, using for example, healthcare ICT-backed, and targeted health information? It costs billions of dollars to treat these diseases. According to Health Canada s *Economic Burden of Illness in Canada, 1998*, the estimated total cost of cardiovascular diseases on the health sector of the Canadian economy was $18,472.9 million (11.6% of the total cost of all illnesses) [8]. This included a direct cost of $6,818.1 million (8.1% of the total direct cost of all illnesses) and an indirect cost of $11,654.8 million (15.4% of the total indirect cost of all illnesses). The total economic burden of illness in 1998 was $159,434.5 million dollars - $83,954.9 million in direct costs and $75,479.6 million in indirect costs. Because $38,266.0 million of total costs were "unattributable", to any particular disease category, although they made up a sizeable chunk, 24.0%, of the total costs, the total costs related to cardiovascular diseases could be a lot higher, and likely to continue to increase over time, hence the need for radical and effective measures to tackle these problems. We cannot prevent people from becoming older, or indeed, wish our seniors away, but could prevent them from having cardiovascular diseases, or limit the occurrence of their complications in those that already have them. Either way, one cannot overemphasize the need for timely and accurate information both to individuals and to healthcare professionals on such preventive measures and progress in medical knowledge regarding the treatment of these diseases. Dr Sarah Jarvis, a London GP and member of the Royal College of General Practitioners in the UK, described the results of the benefits of statins mentioned above as "dramatically exciting", adding, "We have a drug that cannot only halt the progression of the disease but, in the vast majority of patients, it actually showed the disease regress." Professor Peter Weissberg, medical director of the British Heart Foundation, noted that the study was "important," although cautioned that it did not prove that breaking down the fatty deposits would actually mean fewer heart attacks. The study was on patients with cardiovascular disease at centers in the US, Canada, Europe and Australia, who were on intensive treatment with rosuvastatin, known commercially as Crestor, which, along with other statins, reduce cholesterol levels. Some doctors are wary of using high does of statins such as the at least one 40mg pill/ day, used in this study compared to the usual dose of most statins of 10mg or 20mg/ day. The study showed that the medication reduced levels of potentially damaging LDL-cholesterol by about 50% and boosted levels of the beneficial HDL form by around 15%. After two years of treatment, arterial thickness reduced by 6.8%, even more so in those parts worst affected by atherosclerosis, about four out of five patients (78%) showing some such reduction. This study showed that statins not just stabilize plaques, preventing them from rupturing that could result in heart attack or stroke, as previously thought, but reduce their sizes, hence better outcomes of the cardiovascular diseases that they cause. The previous association of rosuvastatin with a small number of cases of a muscle wasting disease is noteworthy, although the medication obtained FDA approval in 2005, and the British Heart Foundation described statins as extremely safe drugs. Costs issues of large numbers of individuals on high doses of the medication are also of concern, as are the likelier occurrence of side effects at such higher doses of drug. Nonetheless, the important results of this study need to reach those that need to use them or that will benefit from them, hence the importance of devising the required healthcare ICT-based targeted health information initiatives to facilitate the achievement of this goal. Would it also not be helpful for example to let the public know how stress can trigger a heart attack in vulnerable individuals? Researchers at the University College London (UCL) studied thirty-four men, who suffered a heart attack or severe chest pain, an average of 15 months earlier, among whom they identified 14 whose symptoms acute stress, anger, and depression, had preceded. Their findings, published in the Proceedings of the National Academy of Sciences in February 2006, showed that stress can increase blood pressure over an extended period, and trigger the release of high levels of clot-forming platelets. The researchers gave volunteers a series of stressful tasks to do, including imagining stressful situations and making a speech, and took their blood pressure, and blood samples for chemical analysis. The men's blood pressure, heart rate, and cardiac output rose in response to the induced stress, and the blood pressure took longer to return to normal levels in those identified as more vulnerable to stress. This group also had higher counts of platelets, cells that form clots to stop bleeding after sometime. According to the head of the research team, and Professor of Psychology for the British Heart Foundation (BHF), Andrew Steptoe, "What's been suspected for a number of years is that emotional stress can trigger heart attack in people who are vulnerable. It is something to do with the way particular people react to emotional stress." Platelets that attempt to stop bleeding when a rupture occurs in the wall of a blood vessel during a heart attack could at high levels, cause blockade of the blood vessel and compromise blood flow to the heart. According to the BHF, "Currently, we can't easily tell whose bodies respond poorly to stressful events, but we can all help ourselves by recognizing what stresses us out and coming up with coping strategies to help control how we respond to these situations." The study also showed that people respond to even stress levels deemed identical in different ways, some more at risk for heart attacks. Medical progress is swift and profuse, the amount of medical knowledge, current, and emerging, intimidating, even for healthcare professionals, not to mention the lay public, neither of whom could ever hope to keep track with the profundity of medical knowledge. Yet, the above example shows how important it is for them to have current research findings, with possible far-reaching implications for disease prevention, treatment, and outcome. These parameters are also important in evaluating qualitative healthcare delivery, and in reducing its costs. Is it not important for example for the public to know the findings of a best-evidence review in the March 14, 2006 issue of the Canadian Medical Association Journal that confirmed that there is unassailable evidence of the effectiveness of regular physical activity in the primary and secondary prevention of several chronic diseases? In other words, should the public not know that physical activity helps prevent from occurring in the first place (primary prevention) and facilitate treatment, and attenuate or reverse the disease process including reducing the incidence of premature death (secondary prevention) of such diseases as cardiovascular diseases, diabetes, cancer, high blood pressure, obesity, depression, and osteoporosis? What would a determined effort to get such information out, targeted, and analyzed to highlight the salient points, cost relative to the direct and indirect costs of the established diseases and their sequelae? Do these examples not point to the need for more intense focus on preventive approaches to healthcare delivery and population health? Would this focus not facilitate the achievement of the dual objective of meeting the core values implicit in the Canada Health Act, yet cost-effectively? Will the resulting improvement in the health of the people not result in even less health spending in the future, freeing up resources for other uses?

There is just as important a need to focus on technological as on medical progress in charting the future of healthcare delivery in Canada. As previously noted, this would involve investing in research and in bringing the gains of research into fruition in product form. Such research endeavors might even be in the more ethereal fields such as nanotechnology, which incidentally is making news lately, regarding its ability to repair brain damage. Rodents blinded by brain damage had their vision partially restored within weeks of treatment with nanotechnology that bioengineers and neuroscientists at the Massachusetts Institute of Technology developed, pointing toward the possible use of this technology similarly in humans in the future. Published in the Proceedings of the National Academy of Sciences of the USA in March 2006, the treatment used extremely small, nano-particles which, when injected into a damaged portion of the brain, spontaneously assemble into a "scaffold" gel. This gel spreads through the damaged area with severed nerves able to grow again through the scaffold, forming new neural pathways. According to a co-author of the study, Rutledge G. Ellis-Behnke, research scientist in MIT's department of brain and cognitive sciences, " If we can reconnect parts of the brain that were disconnected by stroke, then we may be able to restore speech to an individual who is able to understand what is said but has lost the ability to speak." Indeed, innovative technologies would play an increasing role in future healthcare delivery, for example, the new IST project christened OFSETH (Optical Fiber Sensors Embedded into Textile for Healthcare). Applied Photonics Department at Multitel leads the project, which aims to improve healthcare monitoring technologies by utilizing optical fiber sensor techniques in textiles. Presently based on textiles-embedded electrical sensors, the healthcare monitoring solutions OFSETH envisages will instead embed optical sensors into textiles to make the technologies wearable, and enhance monitoring flexibility. There is no doubt about the need for patient monitoring, an important aspect of patient safety, and which would be increasingly critical in the management of patients with limited mobility or who need uninterrupted medical assistance and treatment. This multidisciplinary IST project would enable the monitoring of important parameters such as cardiac and respiratory rates and blood oxygen levels, among others. Sensor technology is also going to be useful in other domains of healthcare delivery for example, in smarter ways to store medications, for example. Another IST-funded project, CoBIs, is examining the use of sensor network technology to enable barrels of chemicals literally 'talk' to each other to improve safety and offer smart shelves that automatically log inventory changes. This project would be more sophisticated than current Radio Frequency Identification (RFID) systems, which in general, are passive smart tags, also in use in the health industry to tag patients and equipments in order to identify them and know where they are. It would create Collaborative Business Items (CoBIs) capable of shifting a significant part of business processes from resource-intensive back-end systems to systems embedded in the products. Attached to sensors, wireless communication and computing components, the products become smart, chemical drums able to warn operators in real time on reaching a warehouse's storage capacity, in the event of leakages, or wrong placement, for examples. This technology would be valuable in the petrochemical industry, for example, but also in the pharmaceutical, health, and other industries. It would be useful to evaluate and ensure compliance with safety regulations, on the storage of hazardous materials or dangerous medications, helping to prevent potentially costly mistakes, in addition to automating processes and increasing efficient operations, with potential for cost savings. As opposed to many RFID systems, CoBIs-enabled objects via embedded sensing, computing, and wireless short-range linkage, actively monitor the state and environmental conditions of the materials to which attached, and communicate their appraisals into back-end systems without human intervention within the project's service-oriented architecture. This makes automatic inventory tracking possible, but additionally sets off visual and audio alarms embedded in the sensors and in the warehouse were it overstocked, or the drums stored the wrong way. The sensors could also monitor changes in the warehouse's milieu, or indeed, of that while the materials are in transit, again setting off an alert as necessary. Besides monitoring drugs and chemicals, CoBIs could create smart clothing useful in protecting workers in hazardous environments, for example, in nuclear power plants, or hospital s X-Ray departments. Several research projects are underway on subjects at the interface of ICT and biomedical sciences, for examples, nanotechnology; multilevel modeling, and simulation of human physiology, and disease related processes; biomedical informatics, and imaging; healthgrid, grid-based health information infrastructure and applications; and bio-inspired ICT, among others. These research areas would no doubt have significant potential applications in healthcare delivery, and influence the future of health services in Canada. Take Semantic Web. This is another of key present research subjects with promising healthcare applications. One of the possible means of delivering targeted health information is via the Internet. There is increasing patient-doctor communication, for example, booking appointments to see the doctor, and text message delivery of the results of lab investigations, and e-mail consultations, to mention a few, going on the Internet, where individuals are also increasingly surfing for health information. The goal of Semantic Web is to enhance the current Web with meta-data and processing means in order to provide web-based systems with advanced (intelligent) features, especially with context-awareness and decision support. These advanced features would include the ability to "reason," which many currently developed Semantic Web languages indeed, offer, although essentially via functionality-based perspectives such as ontology reasoning or access validation, or via application-based perspectives, for examples, Web service retrieval, and composition. Applied computer scientists are taking the capabilities of Semantic Web Systems and applications a step further exploring a viewpoint based on reasoning techniques, for examples, forward or backward chaining, tableau-like approaches, and constraint reasoning, to add to the above features, in addition to being intrinsically heterogeneous in its reasoning forms, as current Web is, in data and formats. There is little doubt that Semantic Web would contribute immensely to facilitating the navigation of the enormous amount of health information currently available and increasing exponentially, by both healthcare professionals and the public. It would also no doubt help with achieving the objectives of targeted health information delivery mentioned earlier. Indeed, novel search tools are making it possible for researchers in the Life and Medical sciences and any others dealing with complex digital data, to find their way through the large amount of raw and derived digital data that genomics and bio-informatics research produce, and to manage extensive collections of multimedia data. According to Les Grivell of the European Molecular Biology Organization (EMBO), project coordinator of IST-funded ORIEL project involved with developing these tools, " Even very simple queries often require complex workflows, involving hours of systematic work in which the relevant databases first have to be found, then interrogated, and tailored to the particular demands of the database s interface. Finally the retrieved information has to be patched together to create some kind of integrated picture." These new retrieval tools would enable intelligent search, able to query distributed resources, interconnect them semantically, and retrieve information in analyzable and maneuverable forms. ORIEL supports biomedical research by enhancing semantic linkages between information in scientific literature, multifaceted molecular datasets and in sophisticated, multi-modal images. Grivell notes that, " ORIEL has supported the development of cutting-edge technology underlying the image ontology-based database of the EU-funded BioImage project and has produced a number of state-of-the-art standalone tools that help researchers explore the scientific literature, and to extract and integrate the information it contains, " for example iHOP (Information Hyperlinked over Proteins) system. iHOP converts the 15 million abstracts contained in the PubMed (US National Library of Medicine) bibliographic database into a uniquely valuable research tool comprising a network of interlinked references to genes, proteins, mutations, diseases and (bio)chemical compounds, is publicly available, and according to Grivell, currently receives about 7000 users per day. Web-based health monitoring technologies, the goal of H-Life, another IST-supported project, is to develop an intelligent milieu useful as personalized health assistant, assisting individuals to select diet plans based on the users' specific lifestyle, medical data, preferences, and habits. It monitors each client individually, providing periodic diet plan changes according to his/ her goals, and progress, all data, and information communicated simultaneously with his/ her doctor. H-Life is also a veritable source of information on health, lifestyle, and nutrition issues, and offers healthcare providers important decision support and remote monitoring of their client's progress. The program would be useful for users such as healthy persons, those with specific risk factors, for examples obesity, high cholesterol levels, hypertension, and high blood sugar levels, among others. H-Life would no doubt help increase awareness of risk factors and promote disease prevention, its key features, namely, intelligent user profiling, plan selection and evaluation, health knowledge bank, advice subsystem and alert and reminding module, valuable tools in contemporary patient-focused, healthcare delivery. However, to deliver on its full potential, both clients and healthcare providers need to have Internet access, the H-Life program with its versatile interface able to provide easy access via a variety of devices, including PCs, notebooks, PDAs, and other mobile devices, thereby facilitating real time, doctor-client, communication and information sharing, including the provision of targeted health information. This program could undoubtedly improve the quality of healthcare delivery, even safe lives, at minimal costs, and it has the potential for widespread use. Indeed, a variety of healthcare ICT is currently in use even directly in the treatment of diseases for example, computerized cognitive behavioral therapy (CCBT,) used to treat depression. Cognitive behavior therapy is some form of psychotherapy based on the concept our thoughts about ourselves, others, and the world around us influences our mood and our behavior, hence attempts to change the former in order to changes the latter. Cognitive behavioral therapy requires the individual to undergo sessions with a therapist, delivered in CCCBT via a computer. CCBT may be in additional to or in place of sessions with a therapist, with the program adapted in different ways to anxiety and depression. CCBT is unsuitable to treat more severe symptoms of anxiety or depression, which require treatment that is more intensive and support from a doctor or psychiatrist. There are numerous other examples of the direct application of healthcare ICT in healthcare delivery, and in facilitating rather than hindering the much-cherished patient-doctor relationship crucial to the success of service provision, and client satisfaction with such services particularly in today's consumer-driven healthcare environment. Patients are becoming increasingly active in decision making regarding their health, armed with information gleaned from the Internet, and with the concept of targeted health information more generally accepted, delivered direct to them via e-mail, or other electronic formats. This ready access to health information helps eliminate information asymmetry, although even in a developed country such as Canada, increasing age, low education levels, technophobia, even costs, and a number of other factors could explain the lesser use of ICT by some, hence the need for efforts to encourage more ICT diffusion in the country. Communication of specific health information could be via "store-and-forward" technologies, wherein information is first packaged, stored, and forwarded to someone for later review, some form of asynchronous communication, for example as in snail mail, voice and e-mail, the latter two, being electronic, more efficient than the first, and increasingly used in consultation, and maintaining the doctor-patient alliance.

Despite lacking the ability to communicate simultaneously, an essential element of the synchronous communication necessary for an ideal doctor-patient relationship, e-mail is gaining increasing currency in healthcare delivery, even preferred by many patients over the telephone. Indeed, computer-based communication is particularly valuable for certain patients that prefer to discuss "touchy" health problems, for example, sexually transmitted diseases, or substance abuse, who tend to feel more at ease volunteering information this way, even fostering the doctor-patient relationship. Not even perennial problems such as privacy, confidentiality, and security, seem able to stop the increasing use of e-mail in clinical work. Security technologies such as Secure Sockets Layer, and Secure HyperText Transfer Protocol, among others, are helping reassure the public and healthcare providers, as are Internet health information sharing protocols as for example, developed and published a few years back[9]. Healthcare ICT is also helping to enable synchronous (real-time) communication and information sharing, for example via live videoconferencing or networked relay chatting, helping to facilitate communication among persons in different geographic locations, for example between patients in remote areas, or dangerous patients, such as prisoners, more efficiently with doctors, virtually "in person." Certain technologies could also relay tactile, "virtual" information electronically from physicians to distant machines that could then enable planned motion. Healthcare ICT is also helping to facilitate self-management of disease, through bidirectional information exchanges including education and counseling, and devices for home monitoring of diseases such as diabetes, and high blood pressure. Electronics health and medical records systems are going to be pervasive standard conduits for health information communication and sharing in the years ahead. Personal health records (PHR), enabling some data entry by the individual is becoming the preferred records storage format for some, who could authorize their doctors, other healthcare professionals, or anyone that they choose for that matter access to these records, in real time. Luminetx, a Memphis, Tenn.-based, medical supply company has developed a new method of palm reading that it expects might even outsmart the other biometric techniques of fingerprinting and retinal scans as a way to perfectly identify individuals. This technology based on an infrared scan of venous blood cells, which a computer then analyzes, Luminetx originally developed to help doctors, and nurses find veins in patients that need injections, intravenous fluids, or blood drawn for laboratory investigations. Although now also marketed to banks, credit card companies and even homeland-security officials as a high-tech biometric identification tool, this technology will likely become more commonly used in healthcare delivery, considering how many lives finding collapsed blood vessels could save in emergency and other situations, for example, after substantial blood loss due to a road traffic accident (RTA.) The technology, which technically converts the human vein into a barcode, could turn out to be an unassailable biometric tool, unlike fingerprinting, for example, and serve as a valuable unique patient and personnel identifier as it would be difficult to reproduce a three-dimensional model of a human venous system, complete with blood. Fujitsu is has also launched its own "Contactless Palm Vein Authentication" system and sold over 5,000 units in Japan, Luminetx targeting sales of its $25,000 machines to hospitals. The technology could detect veins up to half an inch under the skin, using infrared scanners, and analyze the data in real time with a Pentium 4 computer, and then projects a digital image back onto the skin, a greenish X-Ray-like image showing the precise locations of veins under the skin. The concept of targeted health information delivery is akin to that of "information-on-demand" on which IBM announced on February 16, 2006 that it is investing $1 billion over the next three years. The company plans to develop a variety of information-management products and services that would facilitate operations in as varied industries, including the healthcare industry. The firm also introduced a software package that bundles several of IBM's existing data-management tools. The company might want to extend to the health and pharmaceuticals industries its technology developed with Maersk Logistics, to embed wireless sensors into containers of medical shipment to track their location in real time anywhere online, for example, improving a hospital's supply chain management, which could save costs significantly. Healthcare ICT is thus not just going to transform medical practice, but also the business of Medicine, both currently significant cost drivers. IBM is also demonstrating the increasing reorientation in the technology industry of applying software and other healthcare ICT to specific business situations and process improvements, rather than merely developing the base information-management technology, which requires the increasing involvement of professional consultancy services in value-added offerings. In the second quarter of 2006, IBM plans to introduce a product called WebSphere Information Server, which will package a variety of different components for information management, the bundle including capabilities for querying multiple data sources at once and analyzing information, clients able to specify options for managing specific information types, for examples, customer records, products, or identities, cost-effectively. Could some healthcare providers, and any other interested company not adapt this product to deliver targeted health information to subscribers for examples, individuals, doctors, nurses, and other healthcare professionals, or anyone for that matter seeking such personalized services? The potential for healthcare ICT applications in healthcare delivery is profound and just starting, with smart technologies in the horizon that would protect, preserve, and promote even the critical interpersonal relationships aspects that information technology in itself lacks. Again, an essential aspect of the march toward the future of healthcare delivery in Canada is the unflinching appreciation of the crucial role of healthcare ICT in that process, hence the need for the appropriate initiatives to ensure that its widespread adoption in the health system materializes, sooner than later. This widespread adoption of healthcare ICT would require other measures to assure quality, safety, security, and good governance. The idea of healthcare ICT improving healthcare delivery is the primary objective of its adoption, which is in keeping with the goals of patient-centered healthcare delivery. Nonetheless, the patient needs assurance on the safety and confidentiality of his/ her personal health data and information, to have confidence in its use for healthcare delivery. Governments would need to make laws if necessary mandating minimum standards by healthcare providers and others through whose hands patient information would pass, on the safety and security of this information. Such regulatory measures would require an appraisal of the current state of technical knowledge on security at all levels, and with different devices, for example, the Internet, Intranet, wireless/ mobile devices, workstations, and others. These regulations would also need periodic upgrades depending on technological progress, and the terms of agreements between the various technical, and trade blocks and associations crucial to the country maintaining harmonious relationships with its global partners. Much also needs done on interoperability, standards development, quality benchmarking, and auditing of health information technologies, again, areas in which government would have to participate actively. There is unlikely any real benefit in deploying information "silos", every healthcare organization, health region, or province, operating its information network in isolation. Health information could only provide maximum benefit if healthcare providers could share it among their colleagues, and their clients, and access it, in real time, at the point of care (POC). Governments would therefore also need to create the enabling environment for this to happen, as Canada Infoway is currently doing. Even if all government health institutions have electronic access to a national health information network, it would still be limited in its value if family doctors, general practitioners, and other healthcare professionals not working in government hospitals and who are often the first healthcare professionals from whom most people seek medical help, do not have access to this information. Part of promoting healthcare ICT diffusion is therefore encouraging, even facilitating the implementation of technologies, for example, electronic medical records (EMR) and other ICT by these healthcare professionals, including offering incentives to do so. There is no doubt that even with these incentives, the overall costs saving benefits of implementing these technologies, the second key reason for promoting the adoption of healthcare ICT, would offset in time, those of the initial investments in the technologies.

In fact, some would argue that the real problem confronting the Canadian Health system is the problem of healthcare costs, and that the costs issues it faces today are those that it inherited from those of yesteryears. They would argue further that addressing the costs issues therefore is the way to solving the country's healthcare problems, and that although it might seem one-track, this approach would reveal the complexity of issues tied to costs, for example, the different funding models, and the underlying role of healthcare ICT, inherent in any viable solution to the problems. Regarding funding for example, the debate over whether the country should continue with Medicare or have a two-tier health system continues unabated, a COMPAS poll published a week prior to the last federal elections showing that 70% of Canadians would like the government to examine other countries, for example those in Europe, which have a two-tier health system. Most doctors also feel the same way, 70% of delegates to the 2005 annual meeting of the Canadian Medical Association (CMA) in favor of a motion supporting more private sector participation in healthcare delivery. The Supreme Court of Canada also ruled last year that Quebecois could have private healthcare. It seems therefore, that the momentum is in the direction of a parallel private health system, or could it be that this would reverse were the public health system able to eliminate wait lists so that Canadians would not have to endure pain and suffering waiting for surgery and other medical care? Could healthcare ICT not help with reducing if not eliminating wait lists as the example of Saskatchewan recently did, its province-wide Surgical Patient Registry, a comprehensive surgical database that has information on every patient awaiting surgery and their level of urgency made public on the Internet playing a key role? According to a government press release on October 04, 2005, the Saskatchewan Surgical Care Network (SSCN) website updated to include all data up to June 30, 2005, the website, www.sasksurgery.ca, providing a variety of surgical care information such as wait time and wait list data and physician location and specialty. It shows that 50% of all patients wait less than five weeks for their procedures, and 80% receive their surgeries within six months, this "median wait time" information displayed by specialty on the website, for the first time. The data showed that the surgical wait list in the seven largest health regions in the province declined by over 3,200 people between January 2004 and June 2005. That such simple healthcare ICT-based measures as the province took, including accurately tracking and measuring surgical wait lists and patient needs could help reduce wait lists speaks to the immense potential of these technologies in providing effective and cost-effective solutions to some of the perennial problems the country's health system confront. This is not to say that solving the wait list problem is a panacea to the health system's woes. As previously noted, doing so would no doubt ease the public pressure on the current health system to deliver, and the pain and suffering of many that now have to wait long periods for care, but would it ease eliminate the other costs issues weighing the health system down, for example the soaring health spending? Would it therefore, stop the clamor by many Canadians for an alternative health system? Would the issue of funding the health system go away? The answers to these questions would likely be for many, not affirmative, not least because the wait list problem, albeit a major issue, does not define the Canadian health system. In other words, the system does not confront a single-issue problem, but rather faces many interrelated problems that require a multidimensional approach to solving, solutions, which however, the appropriate deployment of healthcare ICT, essentially underpin. Consider the issue of wait times once again. In Saskatchewan, there is ongoing significant investment of federal and provincial funding in reducing surgical wait times, the province allocating $8.9 million in 2005-06, $6.5 million for use to provide surgery to patients who have waited more than 18 months for their procedures. The provincial government plans to target patients waiting for over a year for day surgery, as the number of persons in the previous category significantly declines. Considering the demography of the province, and indeed, of the entire country, it might be more cost-effective, simultaneously, to examine ways to reduce the prevalence of chronic arthritis and of falls in the elderly, the former via targeted health information such as on weight control and osteoporosis prevention, and the latter for which wearable and affordable software programs exist. Would this not reduce the need for surgical intervention, hospitalization, prescription medication, and thus save healthcare costs significantly, and would these efforts not free up resources for the provision of other social services, for example crime prevention and containment? A study published by Canadian researchers in the March 8, 2006 online issue of The Lancet suggest that the use of antidepressants, selective serotonin reuptake inhibitors (SSRI) retard the growth of colorectal tumors, whereas tricyclic antidepressants increase the risk of colorectal cancer. The researchers conducted a population-based nested case-control study from Jan 1, 1981, to Dec 31, 2000, of people aged 5 85 years registered with Saskatchewan Health and eligible for prescription-drug benefit. They identified 6544 cases of colorectal cancer between Jan 1, 1981, and Dec 31, 2000, from the Saskatchewan Cancer Agency registry, which they analyzed for tricyclic antidepressants use. They identified 3367 cases of the same disease from the same source between Jan 1, 1991, and Dec 31, 2000, 3367 cases, which again, they analyzed but for SSRI use, each case matched with controls[10]. Based on their findings, the researchers concluded that SSRI use might inhibit the growth of colorectal tumors via an antipromoter effect or direct cytotoxic effect, and suggested additional studies, with fuller evaluation of confounding factors such as diet, drug use, and comorbid diseases such as diabetes or inflammatory bowel disease. Would it not be necessary to fund further research efforts into understanding the possible roles different types of antidepressants, which are quite commonly used, play in increasing or decreasing the risk of colorectal cancer, which incidentally is also quite common, the second commonest cancer in the country, rates in Canada, some of the highest in the world? Would it also not be necessary to fund research into the interplay of the confounding variables in this context, and to deliver targeted information on research findings such as those of this study to individuals at risk for developing this disease, and those that subscribed to such information besides informing the public in general? Could such information not help reduce morbidity and mortality from this disease and save healthcare costs? Could these findings not have policy implications regarding the use of antidepressants? Another recent research finding that might have important implications for policy formulation is that indicating that the same gene may influence vulnerability to both alcohol and nicotine abuse. This study, published in volume 26, 2006 issue of the Journal of Neuroscience[11], and which the National Institute on Alcohol Abuse and Alcoholism (NIAAA), part of the U.S National Institutes of Health (NIH), supported, was on two genetically distinct kinds of rat. One was an instinctively heavy-drinking strain bred to prefer alcohol ("P" rats), the other bred not to ("NP" rats). Both groups learned to inject themselves with nicotine by pressing a lever. Researchers observed that P rats took more than twice the amount of nicotine as NP rats. The study's lead author, A.D. Lê, Ph.D., of the Toronto's Centre for Addiction and Mental Health and University of Toronto, noted, "Our findings suggest that the genetic factor underlying the high alcohol consumption seen in P rats may also contribute to their affinity for nicotine." Previous research had shown the higher rates of drinking among smokers, than non-smokers, and that smoking is three times more common in people with alcoholism than in the general population. Because previous studies have also implicated genetic factors in both alcohol and nicotine addictions, researchers thought the same gene or genes might influence the co-abuse of alcohol and nicotine, a suggestion difficult to confirm in humans due to the possibility that alcohol use leads to nicotine use, and vice versa. The design of this study enabled the researchers to demonstrate the P rats' affinity for nicotine prior to the animals' exposure to alcohol. The findings also showed that P rats were more vulnerable to nicotine relapse than NP rats and that the P rats' seeming genetic vulnerability to alcohol and nicotine is inapplicable to other drugs of abuse, for example, cocaine, hence the difference between the two groups of rats did not result from a general "reward deficit" in NP rats. According to the Director of NIAAA and study co-author Ting-Kai Li, M.D. "These findings suggest that they may be as useful for studying nicotine addiction and by expanding our knowledge of the genetic underpinnings of alcohol and nicotine co-morbidity these findings will inform our efforts to address those important public health issues". These studies no doubt also bring issues of primary, secondary, and tertiary prevention, as key ways forward in healthcare delivery in Canada to the fore. In other words, efforts to prevent diseases from occurring in the first place, to diagnose and treat them promptly, and to prevent and manage their complications effectively need to intensify, as these would improve the health of Canadians, thereby reduce hospitalization rates and stays, and the need for expensive prescription drugs. Canada spends $4,400 per capita on health, more than what countries such as France, Belgium, Switzerland, and Germany for examples, ranked higher by the World Health Organization (WHO) do, and with total public and private health spending $130 billion and increasing, few would deny that there is a problem with the health system somewhere that needs fixing. The question is why it is increasingly difficult to pay for the health services we provide, which are by no means perfect. Could we for example learn something from countries that also run a publicly funded health system, yet have no significant wait list problem if any? On the other hand, should we be looking at gradually and increasingly embracing private sector participation in the health system, already a 70/30, public/private sector combination taking drugs and dentistry into consideration? Would outsourcing for example, be an acceptable and graded approach to private health sector participation in healthcare delivery that could inspire if not trigger the necessary changes within the public health system that would make it more competitive hence improve service delivery? Would such improvement in services not ultimately reduce healthcare costs while not compromising service quality?

This discussion has thus far deliberately avoided delving into the past of health services delivery in Canada. There is little if any doubt that understanding the past could help chart the path of the future. Nonetheless, historical excursions would only be valuable if not focused on faultfinding. What would the argument be like now for example regarding the consequent imposition of penalties on provinces that allowed "extra billing," after the consolidation of previous legislation in 1984 by the Canada Health Act? Could certain outsourcing arrangements in the present dispensation amount to allowing doctors to charge patients more than the amount listed in the negotiated provincial Schedule of Fees? What would one consider the possible sweep across the country of private health care in terms of the seemingly prevalent province-based incrementalism of health reforms post-major reports that reviewed the financing, administration, and delivery of health services in the country, the recommendations of some of which certain individuals would argue warranted radical changes to the health system? Indeed, some would argue that the federal government should rather not impose penalties or withhold parts of health transfer payments to provinces currently pushing ahead with plans to establish a parallel private health sector, because of major differences in the prevailing circumstances between now and the 1980s and 1990s. Some would add that so long as the provinces do not violate the five principles of the Canada Health Act. The foregoing clearly underscores the need to look back at history with caution, and to focus more on forging ahead with renewed vigor on a new day, with different factors and circumstances operational. Under the present circumstances, with demographics different, disease prevalence and health outcomes, different, the availability or otherwise of health professionals and their remuneration schemes, also different, among others, including the continuing emergence of valuable healthcare ICT, and soaring healthcare costs, should the underlying healthcare delivery paradigms remain what they were two decades ago? Should we be more concerned about those decades-old concepts rather than formulate new ones, more appropriate to addressing the issues of today? The shift from general hospitals toward home-based care and prescription drugs of the eighties and nineties disrupted the neat federal-provincial health funding and administration arrangement that the Canada Health Act had consolidated as mentioned earlier, increasing the expenditures of some provinces on home-based care to uncomfortable levels. Further, some would argue that inter-provincial variations in executing home-based care compromised the ideals of a national health system. With the increasing emphasis on preventive and population health models, progress in medical knowledge and the development of information technologies making them more than self-delusion, is necessarily that on ambulatory and domiciliary care, and on primary care, which in turn means de-emphasizing hospitalization, and prescription drugs, as less people would need them. We are here looking at a healthier populace in the first place, less resource utilization, and consequent significant savings in health spending. Could we avert the problems that a previous similar shift occasioned by making the necessary adjustments to the Canada Health Act, for example mandating service integration via provincial-cum-national health information networks, among others? Would it be necessary for the federal government to create as it is already doing the required enabling information architecture for this integration to materialize? Would it also be necessary for the provincial and territorial governments, the real custodians of healthcare delivery to have their own legislation ensuring the utilization of these information networks, which means doctors having minimal healthcare ICT, for example, electronic medical records (EMR) in their practices? Would the federal government need to keep the injection of health funds to the provinces and territories flowing in order to enhance its influence in ensuring compliance with the Canada Health Act and its modifications? Recent agreements between the federal and provincial/ territorial governments on the terms of the Canada Health and Social Transfer (CHST) guarantee this injection, but what would happen if the federal government could no longer fund this transfer in the agreed forms due to financial constraints? Some would contend that the answer to this question is not so much the need for primary care reform, and to promote health, prevent disease, improve coverage for home-based care, encourage accountability, and use more healthcare ICT. Many previous reports have recommended all these. They would insist it has more to do with whether and to what extent there should be private sector involvement in healthcare delivery in the country. Is Alberta heeding Mazankowski's recommendations for examples, for more cost sharing by consumers via medical savings accounts, and for-profit delivery of specialized services such as diagnostic imaging and minor surgical procedures, and permitting parallel private insurance, or perhaps taking them even further[12]? Would the consumer-driven healthcare model gain increasing currency in Canada, the immense of potential of healthcare ICT to facilitate the actualization of its core principles such as choice of service provision, its driving force? Would this driver also trigger and sustain competitive forces thereby improving service offering and provision, modulating pricing, making qualitative health services more affordable and ultimately reducing health spending overall? Could this be the way out of the seemingly unstoppable healthcare spending increases? Few would argue that no other measures are necessary to solve the healthcare delivery problems in Canada although some would that many could benefit from sensible deployment of healthcare ICT, for example, telehealth, to ease the problems of shortage of healthcare professionals, particularly in rural and remote parts of the country. Regarding this problem, are we going to reconsider Barer and Stoddart and intensify the training of physician assistants, although doing nothing to reduce medical school intake[13]? On the other hand, are we going to increase medical schools funding, or place less restrictions on employing doctors from abroad, or even outsource services for example diagnostic X-Ray services? How could the federal government ensure uniform standards of healthcare delivery under these circumstances? Would it require new legislation to ensure such uniformity? That for-profit healthcare services become prevalent in the country or not, that we change the financing structure and allow private insurance, or in-Medicare user fees, deductibles, medical savings accounts, or not, and that we inject more funds into the health services or introduce stiffer private-sector-style management strangleholds on current administrative structures, would not alter the role of healthcare ICT. It would remain the essential key to progress. The more recent, 2002 Romanow report[14] noted the need to improve the country's health ICT among its other recommendations, many of which the Kirby report[15]that immediately preceded it, supported, but the latter in addition recommended broadening the scope of private sector involvement in a single-tier publicly funded health system. Would some of the changes following on the First Ministers' health care renewal accord of 2003 help spawn others that would guide the country's health system through a new era of healthcare delivery, one with an inclusive healthcare ICT underlay? Would it be private-in-public financing and administration of Medicare, with a mix of private/ public health financing for services outside the core of physicians services and institutional care including pharmacare and home-based care, or more public funds in the latter two, or would it be outright two-tier health services? What additional changes would we see regarding drug coverage? Would there be a move toward more generics than brands regarding prescription drugs? How would this undercurrent of healthcare ICT help shape the answers to these questions? How would government's decision regarding focus on preventive and population health, determine its resource allocation, and could this eventually help fashion negotiations with doctors on remuneration? Specifically, would government resources being more on healthcare ICT-backed disease prevention, health promotion, and population health, including less emphasis on building hospitals but more on strategically placed, centers of excellence, and more on integrated primary care services, ambulatory and domiciliary services, influence such negotiations? Would it be increasingly necessary for government's involvement in ambulatory and domiciliary services, particularly as they would require significant healthcare ICT input for operational success, in order to ensure the success of its preventive and population health goals, which would be critical to withdrawing gradually from hospital-based services, and reducing health spending? Is this scenario already happening with recent developments in Ontario mentioned earlier, or is it with the concept of new complementarity in Quebec? Would this gradual withdrawal pave the way for, or indeed, imply a tacit shift in position regarding privatizing the health services, or having a second tier, for-profit service delivery mode? There is no doubt that although the federal government cannot regulate health services directly, it could by applying subtle pressures on the provinces and territories to withhold or deny funds, or to impose fines for breaches of the Canada Health Act. Perhaps it would prefer to persuade them to work together with Ottawa in order to achieve what essentially are common healthcare goals. Making Canadians healthier is one such goal, and preempts the need for overly health spending. By providing the needed information network for facilitating this objective, it would be much easier for the provincial and state governments to ease out of fund-guzzling healthcare delivery activities that they could avoid, allowing private health services to take over the provision of such services over time. With limited government regulation and guidelines, for example, regarding healthcare ICT implementation to hook up with provincial/ territorial and national health information networks, and issues related to it for example, the safety, confidentiality, and security of patient information, market forces would stabilize prices simultaneously ensuring qualitative, healthcare ICT-backed services, making private healthcare more and more affordable. Indeed, over time, private healthcare providers would broaden their scope and improve their value proposition, offering increasingly sophisticated health promotion and disease prevention services, the cumulative effect of which would be an even healthier populace, and even less government spending on health, resources that would be invaluable in providing other social services for examples education, and crime prevention. This scenario clearly highlights the underlying and pervasive role healthcare ICT could play in the future of healthcare delivery in Canada, including helping to tease out many of the thorny issues that confront health reforms in the country. In other words, it is reasonable to say based on the foregoing analysis that a key step in conceptualizing healthcare delivery in the country in the years ahead is the recognition of this critical role of healthcare ICT in the scheme of things. The next would be to identify specific processes, for examples primary, secondary, and tertiary prevention, and the healthcare ICT deployment that could facilitate their achievement. These measures could be within the context of any financing model as previously stated, although some idea of the direction this and other key issues involved in healthcare delivery would go needs articulating. Because exigencies of various sorts come into play, the approaches to these various issues at the provincial and territorial levels would necessarily vary to a large or small extent, although all would likely be within a general framework in keeping with the core principles of the Canada Health Act in its present or modified form. There are therefore a number of unknown factors among the determinants of the future of Medicare and healthcare delivery in Canada. It is likely however, that healthcare ICT would help in revealing them, in incorporating them in the mix of current variables, leading to the emergence of a new reality of healthcare delivery in the country, a process repeated as new variables emerge, ad infinitum, with progressive improvement in the country's healthcare delivery.

References

1. Available at:
~~http://secure.cihi.ca/cihiweb/dispPage.jsp?cw_page=media_07dec2005_e~~
Accessed on March 12, 2006

2. Available at:
~~http://www.thestar.com/NASApp/cs/ContentServer?pagename=thestar/Layout/Article_Type1&c=Article&cid=1142031015522&call_pageid=968256290204&col=968350116795~~
Accessed on March 12, 2006

3. Available at:
http://www.thestar.com/NASApp/cs/ContentServer?pagename=thestar/Layout/Arti
~~cle_Type1&c=Article&cid=1142031014605&call_pageid=970599119419~~ Accessed on March 12, 2006

4. Chambers, CD., Hernandez-Diaz, S., Van Marter, LJ. Werler, MM. et al. Selective serotonin-reuptake inhibitors and risk of persistent pulmonary hypertension of the newborn. *N Engl J Med* 2006 Feb 9; 354(6):579-87.

5. Yanaihara N, Caplen N, Bowman E, Seike M, Kumamoto K, Yi M, Stephens RM, Okamoto A, Yokota J, Tanaka T, Calin GA, Liu C, Croce CM, Harris CC. Unique microRNA molecular profiles in lung cancer diagnosis and prognosis. *Cancer Cell* 2006; 9: Issue 3.

6. Volinia S, Calin GA, Liu C, Ambs S, Cimmino A, Petrocca F, Visone R, Iorio M, Roldo C, Ferracin M, Prueitt RL, Yanaihara N, Lanza G, Scarpa A, Vecchione A, Negrini M, Harris CC, Croce CM. A microRNA expression signature of human solid tumor defines cancer gene targets. *PNAS USA*, 2006; 103:2257-2261.

7. Available at: http://www.cvdinfobase.ca/cvdbook/En/Index.htm

Accessed on March 14, 2006

8. Health Canada. Economic Burden of Illness in Canada, 1998 (Catalogue #H21-136/1998E). Ottawa: Public Works and Government Services Canada; 2002

9. Kane B, Sands DZ. Guidelines for the clinical use of electronic mail with patients. The AMIA internet-working group, task force on guidelines for the use of clinic-patient electronic mail. Am Med Inform Assoc. 1998; 5:104 11.

10. Available at:
http://www.thelancet.com/journals/lanonc/article/PIIS1470204506706222/abstract?isEOP=true
Accessed on March 17, 2006

11. A. D. Lê, Z. Li, D. Funk, M. Shram, T. K. Li, and Y. Shaham
Increased Vulnerability to Nicotine Self-Administration and Relapse in Alcohol-Naive Offspring of Rats Selectively Bred for High Alcohol Intake *Journal of Neuroscience* 2006 26: 1872-1879.

12. Mazankowski D. A framework for reform: report of the Premier s Advisory Council on Health, 2001 Alberta Government

13. Barer ML, Stoddart GL. Toward integrated medical resource policies for Canada. Ottawa, Ont., Canada: Federal/Provincial/Territorial Conference of Deputy Ministers of Health, 1991

14. Romanow RJ. Building on values: the future of healthcare in Canada: final report. Saskatoon, Sask., Canada: Commission on the Future of Healthcare, November 2002.

15. Kirby MJL. The health of Canadians-the federal role. Vol 6. Recommendations for reform. Ottawa, Ont. Canada: Standing Senate Committee on Social Affairs, Science and Technology, October 2002.

Fixing the U.S. Health System

Retail healthcare, the provision of routine medical services in mall-like settings, is gaining increasing currency in the U.S., with retail giants such as Wal-Mart and Target; regional grocers, Albertson s; and national pharmacy chains, Rite Aid, Brooks-Eckerd, Osco Drug, and CVS, blazing the rail, providing rented outlets for healthcare providers, such as Quick Quality Care, and Take Care Health Care Systems. Such clinics now operate in many states, and charge between $25 to $60 up-front fee, with relatively few clinics accepting insurance, to help with a restricted number of acute medical conditions, between 25 and 30 in all, with no need for prior appointment booking. Interested persons could receive diagnosis and treatment for common ailments, for examples, allergies, colds, flu, bronchitis, headaches, and skin, eye, and ear infections, check their blood pressure, blood sugar and cholesterol, and screen for diabetes, prostate cancer, and heart diseases, and receive other preventive care services. Many have flexible opening hours, including at nights and on Sundays, making them convenient for patrons, which among other attributes, including affordability, and accessibility, has some wondering if the mall or store would not eventually become the first port of call for medical care, rather than the doctor s office for Americans. If indeed, this were the case, would it not dictate new approaches to conceptualizing, financing, managing, regulating, and delivering health services in the country? Considering that new developments are underway in other health and related domains, it seems in fact, that exploring these new approaches is not just necessary at this point, but it is imperative in a continuum of changing variables, which interact with one another to create new challenges. Besides the Solantic organization, that staffs all its clinics with on-site board-certified physicians, registered nurse practitioners and physician assistants, with physician advice restricted to phone consultation typically run these retail clinics, a situation many physician groups object to due to concerns about substandard care. Others see the trend as a way out for millions of uninsured Americans, which some dispute considering that substandard care could prolong, even worsen illness, which would incur more costs, not to mention some of which other Americans would bear one way or another. In fact, some point out the little or no pricing differences between these clinics and family doctors. Would in-store clinics end just being convenient supplements to, and not replacements for, the doctor's office or are they going to play an increasing role with the ongoing shift toward consumer-driven healthcare in the country? Indeed, should the country s healthcare delivery be shifting in this direction? The freedom to choose healthcare provider is the bedrock of the consumer-driven healthcare delivery model, but would the consumer care to be discerning, and patronize substandard care just to save a buck or two? Would the health system therefore be sacrificing quality for choice, and in any case, who are those that pay for the consequences of poor choices? If in any event consumers want to be discerning, would they not need information on which to base their choices? Would they care to task themselves rummaging through the pile of search results before them just to find the latest information on the adverse effects of the presumably safe enteric-coated aspirin? Would it not be easier for them to receive this information and any other health information of their choice direct where they want them, be it their e-mail inboxes, as news alerts, or newsletter, in plain text or as HyperText Markup Language (HTML)? There is no doubt about the value of the consumer being able to choose healthcare providers, and to be active participants in their health affairs. This freedom of choice is a fundamental tenet of efficient market operations, as implicit in choice is non-choice, that is, the freedom to reject a service provider, which engenders competition among providers to ensure the former and avoid the latter. The processes that guarantee the desired results both by the consumer, and the provider, and indeed, other stakeholders whose activities are integral to health services delivery, constitute some of the basic elements of what some have dubbed a new era of healthcare delivery in the U.S.. In other words, the consumer has come to take center stage in the new healthcare delivery paradigm, this position only tenable, given the efficient and effective operations of certain essential processes on the demand and supply ends of healthcare delivery. Some of these processes have always been there, for example, patients have always booked an appointment to see their doctors, and doctors have always communicated the results of lab investigations to their patients, but for the individual and the health system to reap the full benefits of the consumer-driven healthcare, newer more efficient alternatives need implemented for these processes. Could being able to see the doctor earlier or receiving the results of a urinary tract infection earlier not help reduce pain and suffering and save associated direct and indirect costs, for example, of additional medication use, and avoidable absence from work? Could these costs not add up considering not one person but millions of individuals under similar circumstances? Would employers, government, insurers, and the rest of the American taxpayers not also bear some of these costs, to smaller or larger extent? Bob Standing is a native New Yorker. At just thirty-two, he has acquired most of the things he dreamt of as a child, a loving wife, great job, condominium downtown, a trendy wardrobe, and the latest Lincoln Town car. He is on a weekend trip to a rural town in Ohio with a friend when he suddenly takes ill, and by the time he gets to the hospital, is unconscious. ER doctors diagnose him with a stroke, and battle to save his life for hours. Back in New York, Bob recovers mobility on his right side partially after several weeks in hospital and months of physiotherapy. His speech remains slurred and almost incomprehensible. In an instant Bob's life has changed completely, but as we are about to see, the change did not occur so suddenly after all. Bob now knows that he had undiagnosed diabetes type 2 for years prior to the cerebrovascular accident (CVA.) In retrospect, after the doctors told him about it, Bob recalled having more frequent urination, occasional blurred vision, and feeling unusually thirsty, over the years, but did not think much of these experiences, attributing them to one thing or the other, the heat, overwork, and even his occasional bottle of beer. He also recalled that one or two of his uncles died of complications of diabetes, and like him, were rotund. On one occasion, he had complained of severe headaches at work and a friend who had a digital blood pressure instrument took his blood pressure and said that it was somewhat high, but Bob thought the headache caused that and did nothing further about it. The paramedics that took him to the hospital had no information on his medical history the little Bob knew that he was struggling unsuccessfully to give before passing out unhelpful. The ER doctors also knew nothing about Bob's medication history, whether he was allergic to any medication, and which medications interacted adversely with one another, and that he should not take. They had little expertise in the treatment of stroke, for example in the use of tissue plasminogen activator (t-PA,) the life-saving, clot-busting medication whose prompt use could have significantly improved the outcome of Bob's condition. The hospital had no Computerized Tomography (CT) scanner or magnetic resonance imaging (MRI) and had no neurologist, nor could the ER doctors reach one at 11 pm when Bob arrived there. Bob's case, albeit fictitious, illustrates some of the issues regarding the healthcare delivery processes whose improvement is crucial to not just to the success of the consumer-driven healthcare delivery model, but also to fixing the problems of the U.S health system in general.

How promptly and correctly doctors treat stroke are critical to its outcome. Bob might have walked out of that rural hospital a few days later with only minor residual memory and speech problems, if instantly given t-PA for example, under telehealth-enabled neurologist guidance, as the medication is not appropriate for every sort of stroke. He might not even have had stroke in the first place if he had targeted health information on diabetes delivered to him rather than having to dig the information up via an Internet search engine, for example, which perhaps was why he did not in any case. Such information might have sensitized him to his risks of developing type-2 diabetes being overweight or obese. He might have known the symptoms and signs of prediabetes and prevented a full-blown illness, or known that he had diabetes and acted appropriately to treat it. He could have had life-saving even minimal information on his medical history stored in a chip on his wrist watch for example that the paramedics could have accessed while he could still activate access to it even verbally via voice recognition technologies or nonverbally via a number of biometric means. How else could they have known for example if he had diabetic ketoacidosis or was in hypoglycemic coma, and be able to take the right measures, and not give him a sweet drink or insulin, had they thought the problem was the former or the latter respectively, perhaps killing him instantaneously? The ER doctors could have accessed his complete medical history via an intercalated national health information network. With over half a million Americans suffering a stroke annually, how much would having the healthcare information and communications technologies (ICT) in place that would facilitate the efficiency and effectiveness of the processes mentioned above save in human and material terms? A report released on March 16, 2006 on key trends for emergency and trauma services showed that automation would greatly improve ER efficiency and safety. The report, by Health Technology Center (HealthTech) further noted not embracing or delaying adoption of real-time health information systems; radio frequency identification (RFID) for tracking patients, staff and asset; electronic whiteboards; electronic medical records (EMRs) and predictive demand modeling would result in rising operational costs, throughput delays and patient discontent. Predicated on research and interviews with top healthcare ideas leaders and HealthTech partners, the report also noted that healthcare ICT would now, and in future, dictate sophisticated healthcare at the point of care (POC). Healthcare ICT for examples, portable imaging equipment, wireless real-time decision support and video communications would be able to connect say the site of someone's injury to orthopedic surgeons, which no doubt would likely improve quality of care paramedics, for example delivered at the POC, and the outcome of the injury. Furthermore, mobile healthcare ICT and EMRs would help ER and trauma departments manage care by protocol and flow, rather than as by the customary, management by space. Information technologies for examples intelligent dashboards and decision support will facilitate throughput and efficiency, helping to tackle staff shortage problems. Does this report and Bob's case, not illustrate the significant underlying role that healthcare ICT could play in not just fixing the U.S health system now, but also in its future? Few would contend the need of the consumer to have health information, including their own, to which doctors ought to have access at the point of care (POC). There is for example increasing evidence that individuals, even as young as Bob, that have blood pressure that falls below the definition of hypertension are still at risk of cardiovascular disease. The U.S blood pressure guidelines introduced the term, "prehypertensive", for such persons that is, whose systolic blood pressure ranges between 120 and 139mmhg, and diastolic blood pressure between 80 and 89mmhg. A recent study published in the February 2006 issue of the American Journal of Medicine found middle-aged men, and women who did not have cardiovascular disease at baseline, but had blood pressure in the prehypertensive range to have twice the risk of developing heart disease over the next ten years compared with those with "optimal" blood pressure[1]. The definition of "optimal" blood pressure is systolic and diastolic pressure below 120mmHg and 80mmHg, respectively. The researchers found the risk to be higher in blacks, among individuals with diabetes mellitus, and among those with high BMI (>30). Other risk factors are renal insufficiency and cholesterol>4.1mmmol/l, which along with African-American race, and diabetes compared with optimal blood pressure (<120/ 80mmHg) increased the relative risk of cardiovascular disease to as high as 4.10, compared to 2.33 for high-normal blood pressure (130-139mmHg systolic or 85-89mmHg diastolic) and 1.81 for normal blood pressure (120-129mmHg systolic or 80-84mmHg diastolic.) How much could someone such as Bob have benefited from having such information as this? Could he and his doctor have discussed the issue and decided on the best approach to addressing it depending on his blood pressure, if for example, all he needed was diet and exercise, or if he needed pharmacological intervention? Should individuals that have prehypertension, or are risk of developing cardiovascular diseases from it not need to have such information and progress in medical knowledge regarding it targeted at them? How much could the U.S health system save in healthcare costs with the public aware of such information, and particularly those at risk for developing full-blown hypertension and its complications? What would it cost to text message such information to the targeted audience even in an abridged form by say some agency of Health and Human Services Department (HHS,) or to subscribers of a firm that provides such services for a fee? Consider another example. How could knowing about the link that research has established between the presence of the short (s) allele in the promoter region of the serotonin transporter gene, and psychiatric conditions such as alcohol dependence, depression, and anxiety-related personality traits, and that allelic variations in the region, influence response to antidepressants, serotonin-reuptake inhibitors (SSRIs), affect consumer s understanding of their treatment options? How could such knowledge influence health policy formulation or strategizing in a software firm? Could software, based on this knowledge and that persons that have one or two s alleles show more depression and suicidality in response to life events than those homozygous for the long (l) allele, or that more individuals with post-traumatic stress disorder (PTSD) have the s/ s genome type than those that do not help, genotype blood samples instantly? How would doctors receive such software that could help them use evidence-based knowledge as a marker of the likely response of their patients to medications and the outcome of their illnesses in say a clinic or an office setting? Could this not save lives by helping to institute appropriate treatment modalities for a condition with sometimes-tragic consequences? How many more research findings could stimulate innovative technologies in a profoundly dynamic market such as the healthcare industry? What are the chances for new markets replacing mature ones in such an industry and the likelihood for success for a software firm attuned to developments in the industry and using such knowledge in formulating its strategic directions? Would such software not in fact also be doing public good, not just saving lives, but also reducing morbidities, hence healthcare costs? Should government not spearhead collaborative research efforts aimed at developing such software?

Consumers not only need to have targeted health information, they also need to know about the cost of the medical procedures that their doctors recommend, and be able to compare pricing for the procedure with those of other healthcare providers otherwise the whole idea of choice becomes a farce. Here again, healthcare ICT could facilitate this process. A Colorado firm is planning to provide pricing information on medical procedures, for a fee. It is no secret that there could be substantial price differences in the same procedure even within the same health jurisdiction, these differences running into thousands of dollars sometimes, significant out-of-pocket expenses for patients. Many would therefore likely welcome the services of this firm, which announced that consumers could find out the cost of 42 medical procedures ranging from gastric bypass to cataract surgery on the Web site of HealthGrades Inc., based in suburban Denver, which obtains information from 80 health plans covering about 55 million persons. The company intends to add information on 14 more procedures soon. Consumers will pay $7.95 for this service and obtain after providing personal information such as zip code, age, gender and insurance co-pay, a report. The report will contain estimated out-of-pocket costs for individuals that have health insurance; the average price that health insurers negotiate in the region; and the average amount that providers charge and that only the uninsured patient pays. In fact, some insurers, for example, Aetna, already provide their customers with such information, and healthcare providers, including hospitals ought to do the same. There is no doubt that the idea of health savings accounts (HSA) will make most sense with consumers knowing how much a procedure costs. Indeed, the Bush administration plans in the coming weeks to disclose price and quality data from health care providers by posting online the prices that Medicare pays for common medical procedures[2]. The published rates are part of a larger initiative to disclose price and quality data from hospitals, which the administration considers will enable consumers to compare prices at different hospitals and decrease costs. The administration also plans, in the next few months, to post online rates the Defense Department, the Federal Employees Health Benefits Program, and private health plans in six communities negotiated. The Health and Human Services (HHS) Secretary Mike Leavitt noted that government analysts would examine claims data from the aforementioned and from Medicare and Medicaid programs so that "price and quality data will be available for each hospital and doctor". The initiative, termed the "Payer Power" plan, will publish the total costs of procedures, although insured patients pay a fraction of those costs on the Medicare Website. The Centers for Medicare and Medicaid Services (CMS) administrator Mark McClellan noted that it would require hospitals in 2007 to release mortality data on common illnesses, for examples, heart attacks, and infection. Some believe that these published prices will put pressure on hospitals to provide uninsured patients the discounts that they give those insured, and others applaud the move as crucial to make consumers better informed hence best able to make rational choices regarding their healthcare. Yet others contend that ultimately this plan would result in fall in prices and a rise in care quality, as is the case if a competitive market were fully informed. However, some wonder if prices would indeed fall considering as some contend that Medicare does not pay as much as the cost of delivering the service, on the average. Some also argue that increased price transparency should not affect only providers but should also include health insurers and pharmaceutical companies. Others insist that increased price transparency will not resolve the issues of high health care costs and the uninsured, that persons enrolled under group health plans pay lower premiums than those who buy their own health care, and that in fact the plan might simply increase health care costs to individuals. Nonetheless, government is pressing ahead with the plan. After analyzing the markets, HHS plans to ask the markets' largest employers to collaborate with the federal government to influence health care providers to provide pricing and quality information. Health care providers and insurers would need to disclose the quality and prices of their care for 20 of the most common medical procedures for them to conduct business with the participating employers. In addition to promoting the HSA, which over 3.5 million have so far adopted, the program, also will pressure providers to adopt health information technology. Mike Leavitt, speaking at the Commonwealth Club in San Francisco March 14, 2006, noted that pricing information could help uninsured persons bargain with care providers for better deals, adding, "Take hip replacement surgery, for example. It would change the health care world if people could know, before their operation, what the overall package price is going to be, including lab tests, anesthesia, rehab costs, as well as specific information on quality, such as complication rates and patient satisfaction." Leavitt said further, "As first steps toward full electronic health records, insurers, administrators and providers will be asked to use an interoperable electronic registration system that will do away with the medical clipboard as we know it". Is it not indeed important not only for the consumer to have adequate information about the quality but also the costs of healthcare? Would such knowledge not also make them better able to participate in their healthcare, further empowering them, and could providing consumers accurate price information not also help curtail the country s soaring healthcare costs, as competition among healthcare providers compel them to avoid pricing themselves out of the market? There is a clear interest in the HSA, and even with an individual having to purchase a separate health insurance policy with a high deductible, the enrollment for these plans tripled in the past year, the tax breaks clear incentives. However, is paying more out-of-pocket before their insurance takes over for any significant medical expenses, not exclusionary for many, for example the not so financially endowed with chronic illnesses? Does this not underscore the need for such individuals, and indeed, all, to have targeted preventive and health promotion information delivered to them? Does this also not speak to the underlying and important role of healthcare ICT in ensuring the success of initiatives to improve healthcare delivery and reduce healthcare costs?

T o be sure, the issues involved in the current state of affairs with the U.S. health system are legion, but central to them is the increasing healthcare costs and what many insist is the consumer receiving inconsistent, in some cases even not much value for their money. Lowering healthcare costs is of concern at all levels of American government and society. For example, on March 16, 2006, the Democrats in the Nevada state Legislature presented several proposals they say will help lower health care costs, including providing a state subsidy of up to $100 per employee to small businesses paying at least 50% of employee premium, to help fund health insurance premiums, projected to cost $6 million and help 5,000 employers. They also propose to require hospitals to charge uninsured patients similar prices as those charged to insurance firms and to reduce interest rates and fees collection agencies that hunt payments from patients with medical debt charge. In addition, they propose to create Web sites to provide information on health care quality and costs at medical centers and pharmacies, one for example, enabling consumers to compare medication costs at different pharmacies, another, ranking hospitals according to quality data and costs of some common procedures. Many have written on the economics of healthcare delivery in the U.S and on approaches to reducing the escalating healthcare costs. Some have suggested for example that rationing healthcare for the well insured, will not only save money, but also improve general welfare and public health. The premise of this suggestion is essentially that the U.S. health system is awash with wastage, such as non-emergency specialists consultations, MRI for ankle sprain, and other such expensive, and indeed, needless consultations and procedures that only swell healthcare costs, but yield minimal benefits to the patients and for disease outcomes. Many blame this state of affairs on a number of features of the health system, but primarily on the availability of medical technology, in other words that people abuse these technologies just because they are there. Is the response to such arguments then that it was a mistake to develop these technologies, and we should scrap them? Even the protagonists of healthcare rationing would be hard-pressed to answer this question affirmatively. There is no doubt medical technologies have advanced our knowledge and treatment of diseases significantly, but also that their use should be rational and indicated, and not "defensive", for example, because some doctor feared litigation. Here again is evidence of the role of healthcare ICT in reducing healthcare costs, as would be the case if the doctor complied with ICT-backed evidence-based guidelines, which would obviate the need to fear lawsuits besides ensuring rational, benchmarked, practice, with eventual cost savings. It also speaks to the underlying healthcare ICT strand in the multidimensional issues involved in fixing the health system. Thus, government could put a cap on such litigations as President Bush proposed in his 2006 State of the Union speech, a measure that would alleviate the concern over lawsuits by healthcare professionals, and reduce the rate of defensive medicine, hence negate the need to rationalize care on that score. Put differently, why would we need to ration healthcare if the health system ran efficiently and effectively, for example, by eliminating wastage, deploying the appropriate healthcare ICT? Would we in fact not end up providing substandard and inadequate care, rationing healthcare, making people more ill, and ending up paying much more to treat them? Would it not make sense to invest in information technologies that could facilitate healthcare delivery more cost-effectively, enabling us to provide qualitative healthcare cheaper? Could we not alter the present image medical technologies have as money guzzlers via their rational use turning them into veritable money savers? Could we not in fact ensure that the consumer is well informed enough to know the pointlessness of expensive consultations and procedures, and does this not again highlight the need for targeted health information as an important aspect of correcting the information asymmetry that compromises the consumer's ability to be discerning, and efforts to reduce healthcare costs? Could we not reduce the amount government spends on Medicare and on Medicaid by taking a closer look at what healthcare ICT could achieve within the country's health system, in the immediate, medium, and long-terms? For example, what options do we have but to provide health services for seniors? On the other hand, do we not have options to provide these services, at premium quality, but necessarily at the risk of crippling the economy? Should fixing the health system not involve examining ways to achieve this dual objective? Should Medicaid be such a task even conceptualizing its operations and tenability? Is it not a fact that not everyone in society has equal financial endowment? Should we then jettison those amongst us that are poor, or should we find ways to ensure that they receive qualitative healthcare when they need it? To underscore these issues, a federal judge in Bay City, Michigan ruled in March 2006, that pharmacies could not refuse to fill Medicaid for nonpayment of co-pays[3]. This ruling will affect the almost 1.5 million persons that receive, and the over 95% of pharmacies that accept Medicaid in the state. Medicaid generally requires co-pays of $1 or $3 for eligible generic and brand prescription drugs respectively from Medicaid beneficiaries 21 years and older. Medicaid beneficiaries that cannot afford their co-payments will still be able to fill their prescriptions with this ruling, and not just the first time they could not pay copays but not subsequent times as previously, although the state is appealing the ruling. Some also fear that the ruling could result in some of the state's 2,800 pharmacies that serve Medicaid beneficiaries to stop doing so. Is it in fact not inevitable at least for now that government bears the burden of healthcare provision to the poor, if adverse selection would not only prevent them from being able to afford private health insurance, but could make it even harder for government to help them due to the soaring health insurance costs adverse selection engenders? Could we not also ensure that they are healthier over time thus eliminating the screening effects of adverse selection that some argue is even starting to show among employers that now want to be sure who they hire, hence to whom they have to pay health benefits is healthy? Would not doing so not swell the ranks of the unemployed, and place more healthcare burden on government? Would investing in healthcare ICT that could facilitate disease prevention and health promotion not help in making people, rich and poor, healthier?

Besides medical technology, prescription medications also account for a significant

chunk of healthcare spending, but does this have to be the case, or could healthcare ICT help minimize the need for expensive prescription drugs, with $252 billion in annual sales of these drugs in the U.S? Take the issue of heart and cardiovascular diseases. These are quite common in the U.S., for a variety of reasons, many preventable. Boston-based researchers report in the March 22/ 29, 2006 issue of the Journal of the American Medical Association a study directly comparing the effects of physical activity and body weight on cardiovascular biomarkers that otherwise healthy women with low and high exercise and weight levels respectively, generally have less favorable heart health than leaner, more physically active women[4]. This study suggests that women could prevent cardiovascular diseases, including heart attack, the number one killer in women, by losing weight and exercising. Over 50% of the US, population does not exercise to the recommended levels, and 65% are overweight or obese, more women than men, yet, increased body weight and a sedentary lifestyle have significant association with heart disease, diabetes, and even death. This study, in which 27,158 healthy US women participated, found lower and higher levels of physical activity and body weight, respectively, to be independently linked with adverse levels of nearly all of the 11 lipid and inflammatory biomarkers measured, biomarkers associated with cardiac risk and the development of atherosclerosis. Thus, physically inactive, overweight women had higher levels of potentially damaging C-reactive protein, an indicator of ongoing inflammation, and of LDL or bad cholesterol, and lower levels of HDL or good cholesterol, as opposed to women of normal weight, those overweight or obese having 2 to 10 times higher levels of these risk factors for heart attack and stroke. Furthermore, physically inactive women, whether normal weight or overweight, have 5% to 50% higher levels of the biomarkers, according this study, which concluded that a high body weight has a stronger association with adverse cardiovascular biomarker levels than physical inactivity, physical activity linked with more favorable cardiovascular biomarker levels than inactivity, within body weight groups. Could the need for expensive drugs to treat heart diseases not reduce by simple adherence to the suggestions of this and similar studies emphasizing the benefits of optimal weight and exercise? Should the public not have such information and in particular should individuals at risk for overweight and obesity not have it targeted at and delivered to them? Should people also not be aware of the recent intravascular ultrasound (IVUS) imaging-enabled, ASTEROID (A Study to Evaluate the Effect of Rosuvastatin on Intravascular Ultrasound-Derived Coronary Atheroma Burden) study announced at the 2006 annual meeting of the American College of Cardiologys? Published online in *The Journal of the American Medical Association* in March 13, 2006, the study indicated that AstraZeneca s Crestor given at its top 40-milligram dose for two years, not only reduced, but also actually cleared plaque out of the arteries. Other statins such as Pfizer s Lipitor also reduce plaques but none reverses the pathology, which measurement taken with a small ultrasound probe snaked into the coronary arteries showed that Crestor did, including reducing the volume of plaque by 6.8%. The patients in the trial already had a heart attack or other vascular disease severe enough to have them hospitalized, the results indicating that efforts to lower cholesterol should be continuous. With the two-year Crestor-study comparable to the earlier 4% reduction in plaque levels by ETC-216, a good cholesterol lowering drug in only five weeks, which prompted Pfizer to buy its producer, the options for patients are broadening. Experts predict that the results of the Crestor study would benefit its rivals including Vytorin, from Merck and Schering-Plough, which combines Zocor with another medicine, Zetia, to lower cholesterol substantially, reportedly without the muscle-weakening adverse effects of the statins, and Kos Pharmaceuticals niacin preparation to raise good cholesterol, or HDL, which rose unexpectedly in the Crestor trial. Would patients not be able to discuss treatment options meaningfully with their doctors armed with such information? Could this not result in more rational and cheaper drugs prescribed, for example of generics rather than brands, which on aggregate would help reduce healthcare costs? Is healthcare ICT not important in the efficient and effective delivery of this information to those that need it? A number of healthcare ICT for example computerized physician order entry (CPOE) and e-prescribing, would not only facilitate rational prescribing, but also ensure patient safety, which latter by preventing unnecessary medical errors, could save healthcare costs significantly. Even if healthcare providers were concerned about implementation costs and development time, they could meantime implement cheaper computerization, easier and faster to implement, and to achieve a payoff. This was what Wesley Medical Center, a 760- bed teaching facility in Wichita, Kan., did installing an integrated pharmacy automation solution and more than doubled its return on investment (ROI) within four months. Wesley implemented the system in July 2003 and assessed its economic impact in 2003, obtaining an ROI of 211%6. Wesley also reduced error rates in medication selection by 96% percent, enhancing patient safety while saving money, the facility meantime planning for its bigger CPOE project. Crucial to the effort was the July installation of the MedCarousel vertical medication storage and retrieval system along with the Fulfill-Rx inventory management and optimization system, both produced by McKesson Corp., San Francisco. Wesley obtained savings in three areas, namely, daily processing time decreased by 75%; labor savings reductions via halving the time to check incoming orders, and reduction in expedited floor orders by 75%. Safety also improved with pick errors by pharmacy techs that staff pharmacists discover falling six per day to about one every four days. With the "payer power" of the U.S government, comprising 46% of the payer market, it could wield a new kind of public leadership and become the necessary "critical mass", according to HHS Secretary Leavitt, at a Commonwealth Cub of California meeting in San Francisco on March 14, 2006, to move the adoption of thee technologies forward. Pfizer's cholesterol pill Lipitor is still the best-selling drug in the world for the fifth year in a row, with annual sales of $12.9 billion, over twice its closest competitors, namely Plavix, Bristol-Myers Squibb/ Sanofi-Aventis's blood thinner; Nexium, the heartburn pill AstraZeneca makes; and Advair, the asthma inhaler from GlaxoSmithKline. Would Crestor be taking Lipitor's number one slot or would it be some generic from say biotechs such as Amgen that does the same job as effectively as Crestor and Lipitor do? Does the fact that these drugs are the best-sellers not speak to the magnitude of the problems with cholesterol? What does the study mentioned above regarding weight and physical activity tell us about the cholesterol problem? Could we address this issue more cost-effectively as the results of the study suggested? What role could healthcare ICT play in enabling people to know about their options for tackling their blood cholesterol problems? There is no doubt that prescription drugs are necessary to treat many health problems and that government needs to create the enabling environment for pharmaceutical firms to research and develop these medications profitably, for example, by speeding up the Food and Drug Administration (FDA) approval process. For example, two new drugs launched in 2006, namely Sutent, Pfizer s first major foray into cancer drugs, and Acomplia, Sanofi-Aventis anti-obesity drugs will help both curative and preventive healthcare delivery efforts. Sutent is already on the market, Acomplia s FDA approval delayed and rejected as a stop-smoking drug, with some cardiologists, thrilled about its potential to reduce cardiac disease risks also concerned about side effects, in particular depression and suicide, because it works by blocking the same brain receptor that makes marijuana smokers hungry, the so-called, happy receptor . This is information that the public needs to have and that high-risk persons and subscribers should have delivered to them, knowledge that they would need to make treatment choices, prevent unwanted side effects, and which would ultimately reduce morbidities and mortalities, and drive healthcare costs down. In fact, there is much going on in the prescription drugs markets that consumers need to know for them to be discerning enough to make any meaningful impact on healthcare costs. The challenge is to device the means for them to receive this information, rather than to have to search for it, which no one would doubt could be intimidating considering the rate and amount of medical and pharmaceutical information flow. In other words, it is not sufficient for consumers to know about the pricing of medical and surgical procedures, they should also know that of pharmaceuticals and pricing in the health insurance industry. There is for example a silent revolution going on in the pharmaceutical industry that would certainly bear significance for the future of healthcare delivery in the U.S., the war between the brands and the generics, which is pitching firms with over a hundred years history against biotech startups barely three decades old. Indeed, the war is so intense some of the established firms are making generic versions of their brands. At issue is cost, generics customarily cheaper than brands, although often with no differences in their ability to get the job done. Pfizer makes three of the top 20 prescription medications in the U.S., and biotech, Amgen, four, including Aranesp, Epogen, Neulasta and Enbrel. With Pfizer s Zoloft, used to treat depression, and Norvasc, for high blood pressure, losing patent protection in 2006 and 2007, throwing open the markets to generic versions, consumers would also have more medication options from which to choose, at potentially more affordable prices. However, would they know about this development without a determined effort by government and other interested healthcare stakeholders to deliver the required information to them tapping the immense opportunities healthcare ICT offers, for example? Zocor, Merck s cholesterol treatment also loses patent protection mid-2006. The new Medicare drug benefit increases the number of patients using prescription medications. Would it also drive more of them toward the cheap generic versions of these medications, and would that not help reduce health spending on these drugs?

Hospitalization costs also guzzle substantial healthcare funds in the U.S. Here again, healthcare ICT could help reduce spending. Even as benign, a technology as the video game could make a difference to government health spending. Imagine a young man that had a vehicular accident five years ago, and who his physicians subsequently declared brain dead after waking up from coma that lasted over a month, not ever expected to speak, walk, or perform his activities of daily living unaided. Imagine that he proved his physicians wrong in part due to a video game system, now able to speak, to walk, to remember things, even open his hitherto paralyzed and spastic right hand. His parents and experts attribute his remarkable progress to neuro-feedback training on the CyberLearning Technology LLC system, typically used to play car racing video games. Neuro-feedback, a type of conditioning rewards individuals for producing specific brain waves, such as those that appear with the individual relaxed or concentrating on a task. This feedback treatment is not new but incorporating video games into the approach is, and is an example of exploiting the opportunities technologies offer to provide or buoy treatment modalities, in this instance, tapping a youngster's lure to animation and electronics to facilitate and expand the potential of an established treatment approach. By facilitating disease outcomes, these technologies could drastically reduce hospitalization rates and stays, hence healthcare costs. Besides symptoms due to brain injury, CyberLearning's SMART BrainGames system, which is compatible with Sony's PlayStation 1 and 2 consoles and Microsoft's Xbox, is also useful to treat learning disabilities and attention-deficit hyperactivity disorder (ADHD). Other medical applications of video games include helping ill children manage pain and anxiety, games such as "Ben's Game", which a young leukemia patient inspired, and a private island called Brigadoon in Linden Lab s "Second Life" virtual world, helping patients with Asperger's syndrome and autism. Others are Nintendo's new "Brain Age" game to exercise the mind, and "Dance Dance Revolution", which some U.S. schools use to tackle childhood/ adolescent obesity. The technologies are thus also useful in preventive healthcare, which would avert the need for hospitalization, in the first place. There are therapeutic and other treatment modalities for the treatment of these conditions, for example ADHD, including medications, but with parents informed about their options, would they not be better able to make rational choices regarding these treatment options, and does this not again underscore the need for healthcare ICT-enabled, targeted health information? Customary ADHD treatment for example using stimulant such as Ritalin, behavioral therapy and education, often also have health insurance coverage, while neuro-feedback usually does not, information which would also help parents decide on which treatment option to pursue. This example also points out the need for government's continued support for research efforts to elucidate more clearly all aspects of novel and promising treatment modalities, which could prove more cost-effective ultimately, with their adoption more widespread. It also points to the need for a more global perspective of the issues confronting the U.S health system, in particular incorporating a more positive view of the place of healthcare information and communications technologies in its future. The Centers for Disease Control and Prevention launched the VERB campaign in June 2002, the approach, to apply social marketing techniques to the public health problem of sedentary lifestyles among youth. It designed the program to be a presence in tweens (9 T3-year-olds) everyday lives wherever they are, at home, in school, or around the community. It utilized a variety of media strategies, from television and radio spots to posters and print advertising, to a website (in partnership with AOL) where tweens could interact with celebrities and win prizes for being active. Lasting summer 2005, the scope of "VERB" or "8372" broadened to event promotion via text messaging on cell phones. The numbers 8372 spelled out "VERB" on the cell phone key pad, linked tweens in pioneering ways with specific places and events enabling them to become active physically in their own local areas. Could we not have more of such targeted and contextualized health information campaigns now that young people even have more varieties of technologies via which the campaigns could reach them? Should we not explore ways by which we could use the iPod, blogging, cellphone TV, instant messaging, mobile marketing, viral campaigns, advergaming, and other technologies and marketing ideas to target public health education and campaigns? Could these technologies and concepts not help reduce the rising prevalence of crystal meth use and that of other substances for examples tobacco, alcohol, and crack cocaine? Would such campaigns not reduce the utilization of ER services, and medical, and psychiatric hospitals beds, and reduce morbidities and mortalities, hence healthcare costs overall? It is also important to be cognizant of the interplay of medical and technological progress in defining other aspects of healthcare delivery including funding, certification and remuneration for healthcare providers, health insurance, and government regulation and policies. Would it not be necessary for government for example, to establish the needed guidelines, either via legislation or policy formulation that would guarantee the privacy and confidentiality of patient health information for any hope of the fundamental processes of information collation, communication, and sharing critical to realizing the benefits of healthcare ICT on healthcare delivery to materialize? Would fee-for-service not fade out with consumer-driven healthcare delivery, with discerning clientele becoming more active in decisions regarding their choice of healthcare providers and treatment options, replaced with pay-for-performance remuneration models, perhaps with incentives for superior performances, for which healthcare ICT would likely be a key driver? Would government not have to be active in policy formulation regarding speedy realization of the interoperability of healthcare information technologies, via standards determination and policies for their adoption nationwide? Would it not be necessary for government to review on an ongoing basis the terms and conditions of the health savings accounts

(HSA) program based on new data and information regarding the implementation of other programs for example Medicare and Medicaid, and the drug benefit program? Would government also need to review the tax relief offered corporations based on these new developments? The point here is that the factors that impinge on the U.S system might be multi-faceted, but are also interconnected, healthcare ICT the common strand binding them, and a thorough appreciation of whose roles in the different processes necessary for health services delivery, would reveal the required modifications that these various factors would need over time. These modifications are what would enable the realization of the objectives of the country's health system at any point in time, strategic, tactical, or operational, for example, improving healthcare delivery, reducing healthcare costs, and making services available and affordable to all citizens. In other words, having delineated the issues to tackle it is possible for healthcare ICT to help also with tackling them, which underlines the versatility of healthcare ICT in addressing the issues confronting the U.S or any other health system for that matter. It is also important to note the implication of a continuum of challenges that the health system would confront as for instance new data and information emerge regarding current health parameters such as disease prevalence and treatment outcomes, and progress with medical and technological knowledge. This in itself calls for continuing efforts at further understanding the human biology, and how we could prevent it from becoming diseased, and work towards making it even function better in health, achievements that incidentally healthcare ICT could also facilitate as the following example shows.

P hysicians are able to determine what is wrong with us today, but computer scientist,

Astro Teller is developing software that would be able to predict what is going wrong tomorrow via artificial intelligence able to collate and monitor using tiny computers subtle changes on thousands of bodies. BodyMedia, based in Pittsburgh, which Teller co-founded makes armband monitors, 2.9-ounce pods packed with six sensors able to absorb physiological data 32 times a second, the wearer later uploading their data wirelessly to a PC, which transmits the data to BodyMedia's computer servers for analysis by 1,300 algorithms that determine precisely what his/her is doing. The system would learn from data from these individuals to tell for example between walking, jogging, cycling, watching TV, or driving a car, and any other activity for that matter, becoming more perfect the more data entered. With the program more perfect, its applicability to health would become more robust, including the ability to predict when someone will have a cold, headache, epileptic fit or heart attack. It is no doubt obvious the potential benefit of such software for people's health and wellbeing as for the prospects of reducing healthcare costs, among others. Would it not reduce illness rate for the constant body feedback of this software alerting an unhealthy individual to make better lifestyle choices, for example? Could it not enable health insurers to offer better rates to individuals that do not smoke and that exercise and ensure that they really are complying? Could insurers not also use it to price ad review (including upping or lowering) premiums for overweight/ obese persons as an incentive to engage in weight reduction and healthier lifestyles? Would this not reduce if not eliminate the adverse selection inherent in private health insurance, hence drive down insurance costs, while not driving insurance firms which would consequently pay less claims, out of business? Would the overall effects of all these not be, a healthier populace and less health spending, freeing scarce resources for use in other important social services such as education, and crime prevention, which would directly and indirectly also make and keep society healthier? Teller also planned to have an alert system for babies and for seniors living alone. Inspired to form BodyMedia by his doctoral thesis at Carnegie Mellon, in which he set out to explain how computers learn from experience by simulating evolution, Teller s computer then with the help of a learning algorithm, evolved on its own the best means of determining which patients were narcoleptic or depressed[7]. British researchers have developed a biosensor that could warn if a baby has oxygen deprivation during labor. The probe is able to do this by checking for high levels of hypoxanthine, which physicians have known is an indicator of oxygen deprivation. Fetal hypoxia is not only dangerous for the child but also for the woman in labor, who often ends up having a cesarean section if the obstetrician considered there was a significant risk of fetal hypoxia. Because current practice requires blood samples taken to a lab for testing with chances of delay with decision on surgery sometimes taken rather than take the chances of waiting for the lab results, this device could save many a cesarean section, hence reduce the duration of hospitalization, and costs, not to mention saving the woman much pain, even ill-health. A fetus could be at high hypoxic risk with over 5 micromoles of hypoxanthine per liter of its blood. The probe, which analyzes a drop of blood from the child's scalp, could provide the obstetrician almost instant data on whether a fetus is hypoxic, enabling the obstetrician to make more definitive decision on the need or otherwise for surgical intervention. Dr Nick Dale of Warwick, the lead researcher indicated the planned commencement of human trials soon and of the probe's development for commercial purposes. As previously, noted healthcare ICT underlies the processes involved in making the health system work, including the success or otherwise of government policies as the glitches with President Bush's new prescription drug program show. Upon its launching in January 2006, that pharmacies turned many seniors away and could not fill their prescriptions were symptomatic at least in part of computer errors due to the system not quite prepared to handle the increased data loads and other enrollment problems. Seniors with limited budget could not readily switch from state-based drug assistance programs to Medicare and many found the array of choices offered under the program mystifying, although these choices would likely eventually benefit them as they enhance competition, which would reduce costs for them and the government. The drug program, estimated to cost $678 billion over the next decade, relies on private insurers, pharmacies and other health care companies to provide drug coverage for Medicare's 42 million beneficiaries, most of who the government hopes would sign up by the May 15, 2006 registration deadline for eligibility for the program. This example again illustrates the need to implement the appropriate information technologies to facilitate healthcare processes and that it is the appreciation of this principle and acting on it to address the variety of issues pertaining to healthcare processes, that really is the key to fixing the problems confronting the U.S health system. Let us exemplify this principle with the controversy on attention deficit hyperactivity disorder (ADHD) and its treatment. Some experts have questioned the safety of drugs such as Ritalin and Adderall commonly used to treat this condition, in particular pointing out their potential risks to the heart, and insisting that patients and their parents ought to know about these risks. Some suggest there should be a clear, black-box warning for consumers, and an FDA panel's recent eight to seven vote for such a black-box warning agreed with this view, and recommended that patients receiving the drugs should receive a guide outlining the potential hazards of the medicines in clear, easy-to-understand language. Indeed, some argue that there should be some way to warn patients if there was a high level of suspicion that any drug might be dangerous, rather than awaiting definitive confirmation, even if necessary to withdraw the warning if the drugs proved safe. An FDA advisory committee on March 22, 2006, said that pharmaceutical firms should make patients and physicians aware of the potential psychiatric and cardiovascular risks among children who take ADHD medications but did not call for a black-box warning for such treatments as the previous committee mentioned above had recommended. The advisory committee recommended that the labels of ADHD medications include information about the potential risk for hallucinations among children who take such treatments, and that FDA establish a "MedGuide" to tell parents to discuss with physicians whether their children should end treatment with ADHD medications in case they experience hallucinations. The advisory also recommended that this guide should inform parents that ADHD medications could increase the risk for aggressive behavior, psychosis, and mania in children, as well as the risk for heart attack, stroke, and sudden death among those with undiagnosed heart problems. The committee also recommended that FDA should promote more voluntary reports of ADHD medications-related adverse events to the agency s MedWatch system in order to produce more data and information about such problems. Many industry insiders believe that the FDA would accept these recommendations although not sure if it would stick with the recommendation of the earlier committee on the black-box issue. Experts also note that revised safety information labels for ADHD medication might not appear for another few years, although manufacturers of ADHD medications have pledged to would work with FDA to tackle the issues raised by the advisory committee. There is also concern that children who need the medications might not receive prescriptions for them, which calls for striking the right equilibrium between therapeutic benefits and the real risk of serious adverse effects. This in turn underscores the need for relevant current and new information to all concerned, parents, children, and doctors, in order to help with decision making on treatment options.

With the use of Ritalin and similar medications increasing significantly, 2.5 million children in the U.S. taking medications for ADHD, including almost 10% of ten-year-old boys, and over 1.5 million adults on them, 10% of amphetamine users, baby-boomers, over 50, there is ample justification for concern over their use. This is more so considering the potential cardiovascular risks of these medications, among others. Would the health system not be avoiding a potential increase in persons with cardiovascular diseases taking whatever measures necessary to provide the public, and particularly at risk persons with relevant targeted information on these medications? Would the ultimate healthcare costs savings thereof not be far more than the investment in the appropriate healthcare ICT required to achieve this information dissemination? Is the fact that an increasing number of older users, people already at higher risks of heart attacks and strokes, not of enough concern to target the relevant information regarding these medications at them? According to a recent study published by Medco Health Solutions, there has been a 139% increase in the number of adults aged 20 and 44 years using ADHD medications over the past five years, in fact much more than the 82% increase for those under 20 years. Should this not point in the direction of health campaign efforts to reduce the risks of the complications of using these medications? Developing and implementing the required healthcare ICT-backed health education campaign on these medications would facilitate the processes necessary to reduce the prevalence of these complications, and the burden they place on the individuals that use them, their families, and the health system, including in human and material terms. Should we not in fact develop such technology-backed programs that would prevent the illicit use of these drugs in the first place? To illustrate further the need for information to reach those that need them, consider the results of the country's largest depression study that shows that a third of depressed patients who previously did not achieve remission using an antidepressant became symptom-free on using an additional medication and 25% achieved remission after switching to a different antidepressant. The National Institutes of Health's National Institute of Mental Health (NIMH) funded this study, whose findings show that even patients with resistant depression could achieve remission, the patient essentially symptom-free, when treated with augmentation therapy with a second medication, or given a new antidepressant altogether, within 14 weeks. This is the first study to examine the effectiveness of different treatment strategies for patients with depression that did not achieve remission after initial treatment with antidepressants. The first major results of the clinical trial, known as the STAR*D, an acronym for Sequenced Treatment Alternatives to Relieve Depression, study appeared in two papers published in the March 23, 2006 issue of the New England Journal of Medicines[8, 9]. Major depressive disorder (MDD), recurrent episodes of major depression, is relatively common and serious. It could occur along with manic episodes, in bipolar disorder. MDD accounts for 4.4% of the total overall global disease burden, similar to that of ischemic heart disease[10]. The prevalence of MDD in the United States is 5.4% to 8.9% percent and of bipolar disorder, 1.7% to 3.7%. MDD affects 5% to 13% of medical patients not hospitalized, but the condition remains often undiagnosed, but also untreated, and considering that patients with depression are at high risks of suicide, there is no doubt about the need to manage the condition effectively. The findings of this study offer doctors and patients alike important treatment options, but would they know this having to grope around the enormous current medical literature randomly? Alternatively, is it preferable to deliver the information to them? With no significant differences found in the efficacy, safety, or tolerability of the three medications to which the researchers switched the patients, and as opposed to suggestions in previous researches, this study shows that all the medications switched to, despite having different mechanisms of action, seem useful options for treating depression following non-response to the first selective-serotonin reuptake inhibitor (SSRI.) The results offer both doctors and patients the important information that lack of efficacy or tolerance with one SSRI does not necessarily mean the same would happen with another. Should they not know this? Indeed, the researchers advised that augmenting the first antidepressant may be an effective way to achieve remission, and the earlier in the course of treatment, the better, as is prescribing a mix of medications initially rather than one. The researchers did not explore the better of switching or augmenting, a legitimate subject for future research, which may also enable customization of antidepressant treatment to individuals, with even better chances of achieving remission, hence reducing morbidities and mortalities, and ultimately associated costs. There is no doubt about the benefits to the patient and the U.S. health system that could accrue from information such as the above, including updates on progress in knowledge on the effectiveness of antidepressant treatment reaching those that need it most promptly. Healthcare ICT will likely continue to play a major role in making this possible, as a report in the Wall Street Journal on March 22,

2006 revealed. The Journal examined how easy or otherwise it is searching for health information on the Internet, and found that it is indeed, beginning to be easier than before. This is essentially because a number of "Internet firms are launching tailored search engines that aim to deliver to patients and their families more relevant health-related content online". The Journal acknowledged the difficulty that patients could have searching for medical information in the maze that the Internet has become, sometimes even of "knowing the correct spelling of complex conditions", not mention that of ascertaining the trustworthiness of the information obtained. Yet, these issues could compromise the ability of patients to make rational medical inferences from the results of their efforts. The Journal noted the emergence on the World Wide Web of a new breed of tailored search engines that aim to address some of the issues utilizing a variety of searching technologies to restrict the number of pages they search and take consumers direct to the relevant information. Furthermore, some of these Websites organize search results into different categories, facilitating searches that are more efficient. One such firms, is Cosmix, based in California that launched, Kosmix.com, in February 2006. Its engine searches over three billion general Web pages, and divides the results into about 20 relevant categories. One could search within certain categories at WebMD.com for examples news, or even the entire Web. An increasing number of Web sites are using vertical search methods focused on a narrower range of content and able to "pull specific information out of sites to highlight or organize results into categories relevant to their theme", according to the Journal, which also noted that "health information is the next logical place for vertical searches to take hold." It is indeed the case, and with almost 80% of Internet users, now seeking health information via the Web, and online health ad spending projected to increase to $662 million in 2010, the list of Internet firms developing dedicated health search sites, currently including Google, Mamma.com, MedStory, and Healthline Networks, is only likely going to become longer.

More than 45 million Americans were without health insurance in 2004 and the number of uninsured Americans under 65 years increased by six million since 2000. Also swelling the ranks of the uninsured is the fall in employer-sponsored health insurance, by 5% points, with 66% of the non-elderly covered in 2000, but only 61% four years later. Even with public insurance, both Medicaid and the State Children's Health Insurance Program (S-CHIP), meant to fill this gap, there is a significant gap in coverage, as many as 18% of the population under age 65 lacking health insurance, and over 70% of the increases occurred among the poor or almost poor. Employer-sponsored health insurance is sensitive to both the general economy and changes in health insurance premiums, and continues to decrease, even threatening the very existence of some companies with massive lay-offs already at Ford and General Motors. Indeed, GM, reeling under the weight of $10.6 billion in losses in 2005, is offering buyouts and early-retirement packages ranging from $35,000 to $140,000 to each of its 113,000 unionized workers in the U.S. who agree to leave the company, in an agreement it reached with the United Automobile Workers on March 22, 2006. By reducing the number of workers, the company might hope to save health benefits costs, among others, hence better able to rebuild itself as a smaller firm, more competitive against its Asian and European rivals, although unfair competition from which some contend is not really one of the many reasons that GM has been losing markets for so long. Delphi, the country's largest automotive parts maker and a unit of G.M. until a few years ago, also plans to offer buyouts of $35,000 to the 13,000 U.A.W. members of it its shop floors 24,000. Together with the deals on healthcare in late 2005, GM's buyout suggests that the U.A.W. might want to allow concessions without officially tinkering with the union contract for new negotiations. Although how many workers eventually opt for the buyout is now only conjectural, that there is a strong link between health insurance coverage and access to medical services is not, nor that of the link between the swelling ranks of the uninsured in the U.S., and such developments in the automotive and other industries as mentioned above. There is also research evidence that the lack of insurance eventually compromises health because such as individual is less likely to receive preventive care, is likelier hospitalized for preventable illnesses, and unlikely to receive prompt diagnosis and treatment, hence likely to suffer from complications of his/ her illnesses, all of which would increase healthcare costs. Health insurance coverage could improve overall health and reduce mortality rates for the uninsured by between 10% and 15%, and the lack of it, compromise personal finances. The corollary is also true; having health insurance reduces the financial insecurity healthcare engenders as not only are illnesses often unpredictable, hence healthcare expenses, which could also be quite expensive, particularly for chronic illnesses. Ironically, those people that lack health insurance coverage tend to be more ill due to delayed or even lack of healthcare, hence more prone to feel the effect of high healthcare costs, hence pay higher out-of-pocket costs, and experience more problems paying medical bills, than the insured. The question is whether these things have to happen, or are they preventable? Could an underlying healthcare ICT framework help prevent them, help reduce the health benefits companies pay, hence make buyouts and lay-offs unnecessary? These might not be goals achievable overnight, but starting the processes necessary to achieve them now would be laying the foundation for a healthier populace and less health spending in future. It would take the concerted efforts and goodwill of all healthcare stakeholders for this to happen. There is no gainsaying the importance of operational and efficient market forces, even in the health industry, to foster competition not only among healthcare providers but also among their suppliers such as pharmaceutical and medical equipment supplies companies, and among health plans. Even then, healthcare ICT is going to be the major differentiator that would provide market players the competitive edge they would need to survive let alone thrive in the markets. Some like to conceptualize information technologies as commodities now, offering no distinguishing potential, but is it not what you do with your baseball bat on the pitch that earns you an induction into the hall of fame rather than just seen as an has-been? Part of the challenge of improving the U.S health system is for the providers and the other players in the field to be innovative with what they do with healthcare ICT, the processes they figure out, the approaches they adopt, and the technologies they deploy to improve the processes. If high-class hotels now have health, even medical spas, why should a healthcare provider not enhance its value proposition with high-tech preventive care services, for example? Why should there not be competition by healthcare providers to provide the best of such services, or for pharmaceutical companies to develop more effective yet cheaper medications? Dr Peter H Diamandis and his X Price Foundation recently announced his plan to offer, "a multimillion dollar prize to support breakthroughs in high volume and rapid genome sequencing". Judging by the enthusiastic response of scientists to the foundation's earlier offer of up to $10 million in a space exploration contest, which the SpaceShipOne team won, and which no doubt was positive for the future of private space exploration, genomic scientists would also likely respond to the challenge of developing better ways to decode the human genome. This might even just be for the challenge considering that many of the contestants in the earlier venture spent much more than the prize money on their projects. Genome decoding currently costs $23 million and takes six months per one entire human genome. Dr Diamandis reckons, and quite rightly, that cheaper, faster, genome decoding would accelerate the development of innumerable treatments and medicines. Such benefits would come not with having a few copies of the human genome sequence as we presently do, but tens of thousands of sequenced genomes, when statistical analyses would more accurately correlate diseases or drug interactions for examples, with certain genetic sequences. Could these sorts of technology-enabled capabilities not be differentiating for some healthcare providers in the future? Could they not even advance technologically to a level that could enable scientists to anticipate, genomic flaws that could result in even hitherto unknown diseases, thereby preempt them from emerging? Would medical knowledge lead us up to where preventive care would become preemptive care? Would anything be wrong with collaborative public and private sector efforts initiating and supporting such research projects even now, which could mean reaping the benefits in not too distant future? One of the key strengths of the U.S health system is its enviable numbers of high-level medical research corps, both at the basic and applied science levels; one only needs a roll call of Nobel Prize winners in Medicine over the years for attestation. The challenge though is for the continuity of this state of affairs. Is it not possible to conceive a future of a healthy and productive populace living in a prosperous and healthy society and in harmony with itself and its world, the materialization of which such continuity could enable, if not even expedite? Supporting the works of its scientists in exploiting the opportunities that healthcare ICT offers us to improve healthcare delivery is one way the U.S. could achieve this goal. It would then be possible to develop innovative technologies working in tandem with and as the foundation of the efforts to address a variety of processes that all come together in making not just the health system but the society as whole, work, more efficiently, and effectively. However, we could only exploit the technology that is available, and implemented, which is why efforts must also include encouraging healthcare providers and other healthcare stakeholders to adopt healthcare ICT. That few would deny the benefits of these technologies in the health and related industries yet perhaps fewer want to adopt them, or even have any interest in doing so in the future speaks to the major tasks ahead in persuading these healthcare key players to adopt healthcare ICT. Need one say that the continued lack of interest of many doctors and other healthcare providers could derail all efforts by the U.S federal and state governments thus far and proposed, to facilitate the implementation of electronic health records (EHR), personal health records (PHR), regional health information organizations (RHIO), and the national health information networks (NHIN), for examples? How would government accomplish its population health goals without timely and accurate information? How would the surveillance system crucial to accomplishing these goals work without widespread healthcare ICT adoption by the various healthcare providers that would pass critical surveillance information on to the appropriate agencies? According to the Office of the National Coordinator for Health Information Technology (ONC), the federal government has proposed three primary strategies for achieving these goals: unifying public health surveillance systems; streamlining quality and health status monitoring; and accelerating the pace of dissemination of scientific discoveries in medicine into medical practice, but are these practicable without widespread healthcare ICT diffusion? In particular, should efforts to promote speedier healthcare ICT adoption not be a priority if we were to realize President Bush s call for the widespread use of electronic health records (EHRs) within ten years starting in 2004? There could indeed be no trivializing the importance of healthcare ICT diffusion in fixing the problems with the U.S health system and in its future. A major barrier to entry into the electronic medical records (EMR) domain for most physician practices is funding. To be sure, there is promise of some grant funding opportunities from the federal level in the near future no one believes that securing substantial funds is always easy. Perhaps healthcare providers, armed with a well thought-out business plan, should look beyond federal and state opportunities but also to foundations, corporations, health plans, pharmaceuticals, private donors, and others, particularly healthcare stakeholders with likely stake in the practice s success in implementing healthcare ICT. Should a practice not consider for example implementing a system that would improve office efficiency simultaneously facilitating access to patient records, and improving its service delivery to its clients knowing it could obtain significant returns on investment (ROI)? Imagine a hospital that implemented a solution that expands interoperability capabilities and could facilitate information communication and sharing between the practice and healthcare communities linking physicians, patients, and a variety of healthcare professionals and services, via automated clinical and practice technology that is also able to integrate and operate seamlessly with legacy and other ICT systems. Besides its clinical benefits, the system also enhances revenue via improved billing practices and charge capture. Imagine the practice's ROI because of deploying the EMR that reads as follows. $500,000 in coding costs as the practice witnessed an increase in the average level of care for an office visit from 3.06 to 3.26; $50,000 in paper forms and storage expense, a cost reduction of 90%; $110,000, or 75% decrease, in overtime expense; ROI of 40% a year after EMR implementation; and full recovery of initial investment in one year. Yes, these figures are true, with minor changes for a group practice in the U.S. Think of the benefits to the clients of this practice as well, and the possibilities the implemented healthcare ICT offers in terms of improved care, and the reduction in morbidities and mortalities that ensue. There of course would also be savings in healthcare costs that would accrue to the clients and the government thereof, and profits to the practice in terms of increased patronage, as the qualitative services it offers would attract more clients. Such clients might have found out about the practice from information made public and available via a number of different electronic outlets for examples, the Internet, surgical registries, price listing of procedures and of doctors' qualifications, and other practice details. This scenario is another example of the underlying role that healthcare ICT plays in the many different processes that on the aggregate contribute to making the health system work, hence what the U.S. health system really needs to fix it.

P rimary, secondary, and tertiary preventive care should be the cornerstone of any contemporary health system, including that of the U.S. Primary prevention is the prevention of diseases occurring in the first place. Secondary prevention is the early diagnosis and prompt and effective treatment of diseases, and tertiary prevention, the prevention of the complications of diseases and their effective rehabilitation. Information technologies are crucial to the achievement of these prevention goals.

Consider the following. A new AHRQ-funded study published in the March 13 issue of Chest revealed that many inner city adults with severe asthma it seems believe that they have the disease only when they are symptomatic. Asthma is an incapacitating, expensive, and potentially fatal chronic disease common in poor, inner city neighborhoods. The researchers found that over 50% of a sample of 198 adult most of who were Hispanic or African-American that had severe asthma did not believe that their disease was chronic, a common misconception that the researchers termed the "No symptoms, no asthma" belief. Yet, there is research evidence to support the benefits of the daily use of anti-inflammatory medications in improving asthma control, which is indeed, the pillar of National Institute of Health s recommended best practices for treating the disease. The study clearly highlights the need for targeted information rather than leaving individuals to seek it, and for more serious efforts at secondary prevention for example, the need for clinicians to develop more effective asthma management strategies for inner city residents. These measures could be significant in reducing healthcare spending in the long term, and again indicate the importance of emphasizing improving the processes that make the health system work, which healthcare ICT deployed for specific processes could help achieve speedily and cost-effectively. This broader concept of prevention underlines the most important processes we should focus on in our efforts to improve healthcare delivery and to achieve the lofty goals of population health. Salt and fish oil have been in the news lately, developments in both subjects important for the public and of course healthcare professionals to know in their collaborative efforts to prevent some of the most chronic diseases creating substantial burden for families and the health system. The U.K Food Standards Agency (FSA) recently published revised targets set for cutting salt in 85 types of food products by 2010, which incidentally advocates claim do not go far enough. The advocates contend that not reducing salt in the diet by adequate levels could imperil the lives of thousands of people annually in the UK, where estimates show that up to 26 million people eat more than the recommended 6g of salt per day, the average daily consumption nearer 10g. This, no doubt puts them at increased risk of developing high blood pressure, which can triple the risk of heart disease and stroke. Experts estimate that an average consumption reduced to 6g/day would prevent 70,000 heart attacks and strokes a year. Now, is this not a serious public health issue, again, highlighting the importance of focusing on process, this time of the activities of a government agency and their potential effect on health and healthcare costs down the road? Processed foods account for about 75% of the average person's salt intake, experts say. The new FSA targets, which are not obligatory, include: Crisps should have no more than 1.5g of salt per 100g - a reduction of about 10% on current levels; Bacon: 3.5g of salt per 100g; Standard salted butter: 1.7g of salt per 100g; Breakfast cereals: 0.8g per 100g; Baked beans: 0.8g per 100g; and Pre-packed bread and rolls: 1.1g per 100g. Should such recommendations not be binding in the interest of the public, and as part of measures necessary for the primary prevention of the diseases associated with excessive salt intake, many chronic, and significant drivers of health spending? Is this not another instance of the need to focus on processes and take the necessary actions to improve them, including where applicable with the help of health information technologies? In the case of salt for example, should the public have to scavenge medical texts and the Internet to find such information? Is it not in the public interest to ensure that they receive it? It is desirable in promoting healthcare ICT diffusion to aim for most people having a computer and Internet access but the concept of the applications of healthcare ICT in healthcare delivery is much broader. In other words, we should not only consider it feasible to target health information to people that have a PC and could hook up to the World Wide Web. There are innumerable information and communications technologies for examples the cell phone, and the radio, and avenues where we could reach people and use even more sophisticated multimedia technologies to deliver important health information, such as schools, civic centers, stadiums, health centers, ERs, even work places, in intersectoral collaborative efforts. The important thing is to identify the processes to tackle at the various levels of healthcare operations and all the efforts would come together to achieve the common and overall strategic objectives of improved healthcare delivery, cost-effectively. We need to have a vision, a big picture and decompose it, every stakeholder playing his/ her part along the process chain, making it better, more efficient. As previously noted, not everyone likes the new targets that FSA set. Salt campaign group Cash (Consensus Action on Salt and Health) for example, accused the FSA of bowing to industry pressure by in fact increasing its target salt levels in some food categories, its chair, Professor Graham MacGregor, actually noting that some snacks aimed at children would remain saltier than seawater were the

FSA targets even met. According to the chair, the new guidelines would likely result in an average daily salt intake of 8g, not the 6g preferred, "As a result, 30,000 more strokes and heart attacks will occur unnecessarily, 15,000 of which will be fatal." Other critics stress the need for compliance with the guidelines, and according to Paul Lincoln, of the National Heart Forum, without the threat of any sanctions or penalties, some sectors are clearly unwilling to press ahead with healthy reformulations." There is no doubt about the need for cooperation among the players in the matter, including in educating the public on the dangers of excessive salt intake in foods. Underpinning the concept of targeted health information is the continuous delivery of relevant health information including developments in medical knowledge that could change attitudes and practice for the better. Sometimes such information contradicts what we already know, which makes it even more important and perhaps even more urgent to let people know about it. Consider the issue of fish oils for example. Conventional knowledge tells us that consumption of omega-3 fatty acids protects against heart disease and that we should eat up to four oily fish portions a week. However, recent research evidence suggests that there is no evidence of a clear benefit to health from fats commonly found in oily fish, for example in reducing mortality from heart diseases, cancers, or strokes. A March 24, 2006, British Medical Journal review of 89 earlier studies looking at heart disease, cancer or strokes found no proof the fats offered protection, although heart experts caution that we should not stop eating oily fish, such as salmon. Previous researches suggested that omega-3 fats decreased mortality, but the overall picture seems to have changed with this latest research. Experts are looking forward to periodic reviews of research evidence for the benefits of these oils, noting that it is probably not apt to counsel a high intake of omega-3 fats for people who have angina but have not had a myocardial infarction. Other experts are examining whether omega-3 fat prevents cognitive impairment and dementia, while others remind us that medical research has demonstrated a benefit from omega 3 fats in protecting people from heart and circulatory disease. They also note that the fact that this systematic review of numerous studies found no clear evidence either way, should encourage more research into the health benefits, and possibly dangers of oily fish, including why some studies have revealed a slightly higher risk associated with eating very high amounts of oily fish, possibly linked to mercury levels. Such information as above should clearly not disappear into the archives of medical journals, but made available to the public and those at high risk for heart diseases for example, or already have it, who believe that these oils would prevent their condition becoming worse, information that could modify their approach to addressing their health problems for the better. Healthcare ICT is not only playing an effective role in primary prevention, it is also important in other prevention levels, and would likely play even more crucial roles in the future. European researchers for example, have developed an interface between mammalian neurons and silicon chips, a critical first step that would result in the development of more advanced such technologies. These technologies would have important implications for the development of sophisticated neural prostheses to treat neurological disorders, and enable the development of organic computers that use living neurons as their CPU. Although the latter application might be sometime in the future, these new technologies could enable advanced drug screening systems for drug firms, which could use the chip to test the effect of drugs on neurons, hence determine further research prospects and directions. The NACHP project, funded under the European Commission's Future and Emerging Technologies initiative of the IST program, aims to develop a working interface between the living tissue of individual neurons and the inorganic compounds of silicon chips. In collaboration with German microchip firm Infineon, NACHIP placed 16,384 transistors and hundreds of capacitors on a chip just 1mm squared in size, and used special proteins found in the brain to glue the neurons to the chip. However, the proteins also provided the link between ionic channels of the neurons and semiconductor material in a way that neural electrical signals could be passed to the silicon chip, according to Professor Stefano Vassanelli, a molecular biologist with the University of Padua in Italy, and one of the partners in the project. The chip's transistors then record the arriving signals. It is also possible to stimulate the neurons via the capacitors, enabling two-way communications. The researchers continue to work on improving methods of stimulating the neurons without causing any damage to them, and on how to communicate with the neurons via genes, and to explore ways to utilize genes to control the neuro-chip, and develop a genetically powered hard disk. These future research efforts would no doubt require multidisciplinary collaboration perhaps even across continents, efforts that could dramatically change healthcare delivery for the better, including reducing healthcare costs on the chronic and debilitating diseases that many neurological diseases for example, are. Investing in healthcare ICT now both at the research and product development levels could therefore also be valuable in secondary and tertiary prevention as the above example shows, capable of reducing the costs of neuron-rehabilitation, and not just of the immediate treatment of neurological conditions, both significant sources of health burden on the individuals affected, their families, and society. The example of physicians with Michigan's Henry Ford Medical Group that recently took part in an e-prescribing project illustrates how healthcare ICT could help save significant healthcare costs. The physicians wrote over 500,000 prescriptions electronically during the project, improving the use of generic medications by 7.3%. They saved $3.1 million in pharmacy costs over a one-year period. The 800-member practice now has 300 doctors at 24 medical centers who prescribe electronically. Other highlights of the project include changing or cancelling over 50,000 prescriptions after the system alerted users to medications that were on the formulary. This increased the use of generic drugs, contributing to overall costs savings. Furthermore, the change or cancellation of over 80,000 prescriptions due to alerts for drug-to-drug interactions no doubt significantly contributed to patient safety, also saving costs that might have accrued from attendant morbidities and mortalities, otherwise. The 60-doctor e-prescribing project commenced in 2005, via the Henry Ford Medical Group and Health Alliance Plan, and was part of a larger Southeast Michigan e-Prescribing Initiative from General Motors, Ford Motor Company, DaimlerChrysler, Michigan health plans and pharmacy benefit manager Medco Health Solutions. There is no doubt that with many more healthcare providers embracing e-prescribing, its potential for improving healthcare delivery and saving healthcare costs would become increasingly manifest. Examples of healthcare information and communications technologies deployed to address clinical and public health processes abound, as do of those that aim to improve administrative and management processes in the health industry. The key is to recognize the potential of these technologies in improving the many processes that operate to make the health system function more efficiently and effectively, and capitalize on the opportunities these technologies, current and emerging, offer to improve the health system. This way, we could fix the U.S. health system, assure access to qualitative and affordable healthcare delivery, and significantly reduce health spending without compromising the quality of the services delivered.

References

1. Kshirsagar AV, Carpenter M, Bang H, Wyatt SB, Colindres RE. Blood Pressure Usually Considered Normal Is Associated with an Elevated Risk of Cardiovascular Disease February 2006, Pages 133-141

2. Available at:
http://www.detnews.com/apps/pbcs.dll/article?AID=/20060317/LIFESTYLE03/603170322&SearchID=73238742221807
Accessed on March 21, 2006

3. Available at:
http://www.kaisernetwork.org/daily_reports/rep_index.cfm?hint=3&DR_ID=36083
Accessed on March 21, 2006

4. Mora, S, Lee, I-Min, Buring, JE, Ridker, PM. Association of Physical Activity and Body Mass Index with Novel and Traditional Cardiovascular Biomarkers in Women. *JAMA*. 2006; 295:1412-1419.

5. Nissen SE, Nicholls SJ, Sipahi I, et al. Effect of very high-intensity statin therapy on regression of coronary atherosclerosis: the ASTEROID trial. *JAMA*. 2006; 295 :(doi:10.1001/jama.295.13.jpc60002).

6. Available at: http://www.healthcareitnews.com/story.cms?id=703
Accessed on March 22, 2006

7. Available at: http://www.forbes.com/free_forbes/2005/0606/071.html
Accessed on March 22, 2006

8. Rush, A. J., Trivedi, M. H., Wisniewski, S. R., Stewart, J. W., Nierenberg, A. A., Thase, M. E., Ritz, L., Biggs, M. M., Warden, D., Luther, J. F., Shores-Wilson, K.,

Niederehe, G., Fava, M., the STAR*D Study Team, (2006). Bupropion-SR, Sertraline, or Venlafaxine-XR after Failure of SSRIs for Depression. *NEJM* 354: 1231-1242

9. Trivedi, M. H., Fava, M., Wisniewski, S. R., Thase, M. E., Quitkin, F., Warden, D., Ritz, L., Nierenberg, A. A., Lebowitz, B. D., Biggs, M. M., Luther, J. F., Shores-Wilson, K., Rush, A. J., the STAR*D Study Team, (2006). Medication Augmentation after the Failure of SSRIs for Depression. *NEJM* 354: 1243-1252

10. Mann JJ. The Medical Management of Depression. *NEJM.* Vol. 353:1819-1834, October 27, 2005

11. Available at: http://www.medicalnewstoday.com/medicalnews.php?newsid=40011# Accessed on March 23, 2006

12. BMJ, doi:10.1136/bmj.38798.680185.47 (published 24 March 2006) Copyright March 24, 2006

Conclusion

The increasing prevalence of chronic health problems, for example, obesity and its associated diseases, is a major healthcare costs driver in the three countries we here consider. Obesity rates are reaching almost epidemic proportions with experts warning that this trend could negate any health gains that these countries make now, and in future, which would worsen the burden of disability and, although perhaps more than reduce life expectancy. An aging population, in the U.S., those 85 years and older, the fastest-growing age group, about 1% of the population, compared with about 0.1% in 1900, would likely increase the number of patients with Alzheimer's disease, which already costs the U.S. for example, about $100 billion annually. Indeed, because people are living longer, although not necessarily free of disease, but are not working longer, programs such as Medicare in the U.S and Canada, and the NHS in the U.K, will likely face future budgetary issues. The increasing use of mind-altering substances, licit, for example, alcohol, and illicit, for example, crystal meth, will contribute to likely increase the prevalence of chronic diseases, escalating the already troubling excessive health spending in these countries. Recent surveys show that about a quarter of seniors aged 75 years and over, in the U.S. visit hospital emergency rooms (ER) at least four times a year, a quarter, actually 10 or more times. Furthermore, for each dollar spent on health care for U.S. seniors, Medicare, and Medicaid fund 65 cents, patients out-of-pocket spending 19 cents, and private insurance, 12cents hence government bears most of their healthcare costs. With almost 80% of U.S, seniors having at least one chronic illness and about 50% at least two, and obesity rates in this age group increasing, about 33% of senior men and 39% of senior women obese, they are likely to continue to incur significant healthcare costs, but should they? Could we not reduce the prevalence of obesity and chronic diseases among seniors via healthcare ICT-backed targeted health information and other health campaign programs? Could we not reduce the prevalence of falls for example among seniors if they wore software programs that could warn them about and prevent an imminent fall, or with which they could seek help if they lived alone, facilitating access to healthcare and minimizing possible complications? Would this not reduce the burden of hip and other fractures in this vulnerable population and reduce healthcare costs? Could we via the effective utilization of healthcare ICT not facilitate the ambulatory and domiciliary management of the health problems of seniors thereby not only enabling them to receive care in the comfort of their homes and among their loved ones, but also reducing hospitalization rates and stays, hence healthcare costs overall? Would these measures not help reduce healthcare costs in the U.K, and Canada, with similar healthcare delivery issues pertaining to their seniors, differences in health funding systems in these countries regardless?

Some experts contend that the effect of aging baby boomers on Medicare and the government in the U.S. might not be as large as previously thought because today's seniors compared to those even just two decades ago are showing considerably less disability, regardless of gender. Extrapolated forward, this suggests that tomorrow's seniors would show even less disability, provided of course we consolidate rather than lose the gains made. On the surface, it should be easy to consolidate the gains, but what should we make of the increasing prevalence of obesity for example, and does it not portend possible increases in its associated chronic diseases? Are these Americans not those that will become seniors someday? What health problems are they nurturing now being so obese that they would take with them into later life and what would the effect of this be on the nation's fiscal health? Should we not intensify efforts to use whatever applicable multimedia health information technologies we could to target important health information to those that need them, rather than hope that they would seek the information themselves? Even if they did, could the frustration of the difficulties accessing relevant information via Internet search engines for example, be the reason many do not know the health risks of some of their unhealthy habits? Could it be that people respond better to health information targeted in particular ways, for example contextually to appeal to certain groups of people? Should our efforts at changing peoples' attitude to health information not therefore focus on these considerations? Would the efforts not be worthwhile considering the issues at stake, for example, the prospects of a future generation of seniors unhealthier than those of today? Would doing nothing about today's obesity of tomorrow's seniors not be reversing the gains we seem to be making now? What considerations should override investing in healthcare information and communications technologies if their deliberate and appropriate deployment could help avert this reversal? What are the chances that programs such as the Medicare drug benefit program would achieve its goals without efficient health information technologies to facilitate the various processes involved in making it work, as its reported glitches when launched recently showed? Even if the U.S. federal government continues to increase the health savings accounts (HSA) and modify federal tax laws that some contend essentially encourage workers to yield control over their health care to their employers, which translates to losing their health insurance post-employment, would people not even need to know what HSA means? These examples show the importance of information flow regarding whatever process involved in making the health system works. Increasing the HSA would enable a worker to buy preferred coverage than employer-imposed, for example, also able to keep it even post-employment. The higher HSAs are, the likelier also the achievement of one of the key goals of consumer-driven healthcare, that of increased competition among insurers, thereby making health care more affordable for workers unable to have coverage, because they are too ill or poor. However, would the consumer be able to make rational choices that would foster such competition not armed with the necessary information to facilitate that judgment? The point here is that healthcare delivery is an assortment of processes. Many of the problems health systems in these countries currently face are traceable to flaws in these processes, hence the need to embrace and implement healthcare ICT, in order to rectify these flaws. Few would argue for example, that improving accountability among NHS Trusts could not benefit from automation of the some of the processes of these health organizations, or that health regions in Canada could not fare better with faster, more efficient processes in their administrative, and management, not to mention their clinical domains.

There is no doubt that some regulating but not over-regulating would make the

health systems in these countries work better. One reason for the slow adoption of healthcare ICT is concern over the privacy and confidentiality of health information. These are genuine concerns that not only require standards to which all healthcare stakeholders involved with handling and sharing such information should comply, but which in fact might require legislative teeth to enforce such compliance. Considering that realizing the full benefits of these technologies, including reducing overall healthcare costs eventually, requires information flow for example the available of timely and accurate health information of patients at the point of care (POC), the need for such legislation should defy contention. Nonetheless, there are other kinds of legislation that could actually hinder the achievements of the goals of reducing healthcare costs, such as, excessive regulation by the states, some of which even bar people from buying insurance from carriers in another state, such state regulations estimated to increase insurance premiums by up to 15%. Besides such regulations, defeat the concept of promoting competition among carriers, and the entire idea of consumer-driven healthcare. However, even scrapping those regulations, which should enable consumers buy insurance in states with lower regulatory costs, would still not facilitate interstate business activities without the necessary technology infrastructure in place for seamless patient information communication and sharing. This again emphasizes the need for such technologies to improve the processes necessary to make health systems work more efficiently, which is what would really reduce healthcare costs.

The discussion thus far clearly focuses on what we could achieve reducing healthcare costs without compromising healthcare quality using healthcare ICT. Some admit that the intent of the U.S Medicare drug program, for example, to achieve more health coverage is noble, but that it has made many lose coverage, but should it be doing that? Would more efficient deployment of healthcare information technologies to improve the processes associated with the program's implementation, not rectify the problems it had on launching? Does that mean that government should scrap the program? There is no doubt that there are numerous administrative, legal, tax, and other approaches to helping fix the healthcare problems in these three countries, but it would become clear on scrutiny that it is possible to decompose these issues into intercalated processes that need continuing reappraisals and the deployment of appropriate information technologies to improve. With improvement will come cost reduction, some, much like all the other benefits derivable from implementing these technologies, immediate, others medium-, yet, others even long-term. However, with measured expectations of achievable objectives, we could all be rest assured that the problems health systems in these, and other countries confront are solvable, even preventable, via the implementation of appropriate, process-oriented, healthcare ICT.

Copyright Bankix Systems Ltd March 25, 2006

www.ingramcontent.com/pod-product-compliance
Lightning Source LLC
Chambersburg PA
CBHW030706220526
45463CB00005B/1925